The Ketogenic Key:

Unlock the Secrets to Lose Weight, Slow Aging, Stop Inflammation, and Prevent Disease!

Lori Shemek, PhD, CNC and Steve Welch, CFNC

The Ketogenic Key

First Printing, published July 2020
Copyright © Lori Shemek and Steve Welch, 2020
All Rights Reserved

LIBRARY OF CONGRESS CATALOGING-IN-PUBLICATION DATA
The Ketogenic Key: Unlocking the Secrets to Lose Weight, Slow Aging, Stop Inflammation, and Prevent Disease!
Shemek, Lori
Welch, Steve
ISBN: 978-1-7350553-0-5

Disclaimer

The ideas, concepts, opinions, nutrition recommendations, and exercise techniques expressed and discussed in this book are those of the authors, except where otherwise noted, and are intended to be used for educational purposes only. All efforts have been made to ensure that the information contained in this book is accurate and up to date. This book is provided with the understanding that the authors and publisher are not prescribing medical advice of any kind. The information contained within this book is not intended to be used as medical advice or replace medical advice for the treatment of any disease, condition, illness, or injury. Before beginning any nutrition and/or exercise program, it is imperative that any individual first consult with and receive full medical clearance from a licensed physician or healthcare provider. The authors and publisher disclaim responsibility and are not liable to any person or entity for damage, injury, or medical outcomes that occur or alleged to be directly or indirectly resulting from the application or interpretation of any information, material, or methods described or displayed in this book.

Acknowledgements

Lori and Steve are indebted to the insightful and sage Bob Choat for his guidance and ideas during the development of this book, as well as the talented Lisa Klein of Pisa Design for the stunning book cover.

Dedications

I lovingly commit this work to all individuals who need proof that they are not an exception – optimal health is absolutely possible for you, too.
~Lori

To JD Griffin and James Rice, if it weren't for the two of you starting me on the low-carb and then keto path, this book would not exist. And to my parents (RIP Mom), thank you for teaching and encouraging me to think critically, research information, and to investigate that about which I am curious. I know you're shocked that my first book isn't about dinosaurs or giant squids.
~Steve

Here's What Other Authors and Experts Are Saying About *The Ketogenic Key:*

"This ground-breaking book, *The Ketogenic Key*, is so much more than just another keto diet and recipe book. The authors leave no stone unturned as they demystify ketosis, and give you simple, clear info about why ketosis works so well, how it can improve multiple aspects of your health and well-being, and a step-wise approach that shows how you can get the benefits of ketosis, with and without strict dieting! This is a must-read for anyone who is keto-curious!"
— JJ Virgin, best-selling author of *JJ Virgin's Sugar Impact Diet*

"*The Ketogenic Key* is a powerful and compelling read backed by science! If you want a book that delivers sound advice, busts many myths and misconceptions about the ketogenic diet, and explores other techniques to optimize and maintain ketosis, then this is the book for you."
— Dr. James DiNicolantonio, Cardiovascular Research Scientist and author of *The Salt Fix*, *Superfuel*, and *The Longevity Solution*

"As host of a syndicated health radio show for 20 years, I've had the honor of interviewing **all** of today's leading diet and nutrition experts. I've also read their books. Dr. Shemek's *The Ketogenic Key* is the most simplified and informative book ever written on the topic! She busts all the keto myths and gives you the *key* to unlock your genetic potential, reach your ideal weight, and achieve optimal health."
— Dr. David Friedman, international award-winning, #1 best-selling author of *Food Sanity*

"*The Ketogenic Key* is a preeminent guide for all things keto. Lori Shemek brilliantly breaks down the benefits of going keto for various health problems, common myths and misconceptions, and how to get started, along with delicious recipes and game-changing tips to take your keto journey to the next level. If you have ever been interested in starting keto but been putting it off, *The Ketogenic Key* is the book you need to help you not only get started but thrive with this new way of eating."
— Dr. Will Cole, leading functional medicine expert and best-selling author, *The Inflammation Spectrum* and *Ketotarian*

"Lori Shemek and Steve Welch do a great job of covering everything you need to know about ketosis, and they do it in an easy to understand way."
— Maria Emmerich, international best-selling author of *Keto: The Complete Guide to Success on the Keto Diet*

Table of Contents

Section V: Getting Started With and Maintaining *The Ketogenic Key* Lifestyle   **140**

Section VI: What to Eat, What Not to Eat, Shopping Lists and Recipes   **175**

Section VII: The Ketogenic Key – Concluding Thoughts   **258**

Section VIII: Selected Annotated References and Summaries   **260**

Author Profiles   **314**

ABOUT THE AUTHORS

Lori Shemek, PhD, CNC

I grew up with a single mother who did not feel she had many choices in life, nor did she believe she deserved health and happiness. Consequently, my wonderful mother created a challenging life for herself. She was understandably, chronically stressed; we had little to no money; no support from family or my father as he was missing from the picture. She smoked heavily, her diet was highly processed with a personal emphasis on sugar, she was very overweight, and suffered from a myriad of health conditions. In fact, most of the memories I have of my sweet mother are of her not well, suffering.

As a child, I was always interested in health and I knew her choices were affecting her greatly. I remember often, just walking into her room seeing her laying there in the dark suffering, and it broke my heart but I knew, intuitively, she could make different choices. I also remember struggling to create a healthier lifestyle for myself and my two younger brothers, whose care was often left to me.

My mother died at the young age of thirty-six, leaving behind 3 young children with literally nowhere to go. It was at my mother's memorial service that I had an *"aha!"* moment where I vividly remember saying to myself: *She didn't have to die. She could have made different choices!* It was right then, I decided what I wanted to do with my life: I wanted to help people make healthier choices and know they do have choices to make.

My journey has been an interesting one. I finished high school, and focused on finding a way to get to college. After earning my Ph.D. in psychology, I got a job as a casework therapist for a nonprofit in Dallas dedicated to the prevention of child abuse and neglect - eventually becoming vice-president of the organization. But as committed as I was to the emotional well being of our clients, I never let go of my interest in diet and health. When I would meet with my clients, I couldn't help but notice how poorly some of them were eating. I began creating nutritional plans for families that would include giving up sugar and soda and introducing veggies and other healthful foods. When the clients began following my advice, we could all see the improvements in their lives in very dramatic ways. My work allowed me to see firsthand the extent to which physical health seriously impacts emotional health and vice versa. It was becoming more apparent to me that I needed to find a way to fulfill my lifelong interest in nutrition and health, so I left my job to create a business that would help others optimize their health and weight. My goal was to marry my background in psychology, with my strong commitment to nutrition and health. With that in mind, I went back to school and earned my Certification in Nutritional Counseling and also became a Certified Life Coach to create my own health coaching company called DLS HealthWorks, LLC.

My personal dream and passion is to help as many people as possible to achieve more satisfying lives. I want to support people with health, weight and mindset issues to create positive change and alter the way they view themselves in relation to the world. I want them to realize that they have greater control and always have the option of making different choices. My mission and passion is to guide women and men to change their health and life where they not only feel healthy, but also an improved sense of self-worth. My sincere desire has been in creating global awareness of low-level inflammation and how it is responsible for the core, underlying cause of most illness, disease, faster aging and weight gain. Ketosis specifically impacts mechanisms responsible for chronic inflammation.

This mission has been an ever-winding path that has allowed me to help fulfill my passion of helping others.

I have authored three prior best-selling books all dedicated to helping my readers; clients and followers change their health and weight. I have also had the opportunity to share my work via the major media outlets such as television, radio, podcasts, speaking and of course, my books.

This book you are holding in your hand is an exceptional work that is science-based with in-depth annotated research. Steve Welch,

About the Authors

my co-author, is a medical writer and researcher who I believe has added such quality information, information that is rare to find elsewhere. Steve and I worked together on this book tirelessly for over a year and we are very proud of it! We actually kept delaying it due to new research coming in.

It's important to understand that research has shown us how powerful ketosis is – that is truly the *key* to optimizing your health, weight, brain health, mental well being, gut health and much more.

So let's get started!

Lori L. Shemek, PhD, CNC

Stephen (Steve) Welch, CFNC

What gives a former non-profit medical society senior executive, publisher, and CEO the credentials and desire to help a celebrity health, nutrition, and fitness expert like Dr. Lori Shemek write a book about ketogenic therapies? The short answer is, life changing personal experience! *I am a living, breathing, ketone-powered example of how this lifestyle can improve multiple aspects of your life, and because of this, I am passionate about sharing the secrets of The Ketogenic Key with everyone.*
In addition, while writing this book, I studied for and passed my exam to get my credentials as a NESTA Certified Fitness Nutrition Coach, to further augment my ability to help others achieve their goals.

I'll get right to the point. I have "been there, done that" in terms of being unhealthy, needing to lose weight, and taking action to make it happen.

Here's how my ketogenic journey started: in 2013, I was about 35-40 pounds overweight. I knew I had gained some weight over recent years, primarily from not watching my diet and indulging in too many nice foodie dinners with plenty of rich foods, primo wine, and decadent desserts. At the time, I just thought I was treating myself, and deserved to eat what I wanted, after all, I worked hard, played hard, and I was exercising pretty regularly. Yet, my weight crept up and my pants kept getting tighter. My running internal monologue joke was that the dry cleaner shrunk my suit pants again.

The reality check hit smacked me in the face in October of 2013. I worked for a global medical membership and education organization called the American College of Chest Physicians. We were holding our annual international conference, where about 5,000 doctors from all over the world would attend and hear the latest research and therapeutic lung disease information for the fields of pulmonary and critical care medicine. About 10 years prior, I had traveled to China to help launch a Chinese language edition of our medical journal, *CHEST*. At the meeting in 2013, I ran into Dr. Sunny, one of the Chinese physicians I had met in 2003. She immediately looked me up and down and said, "Oh, I can tell you have become VERY successful!" I looked at her with a puzzled, wrinkled brow and said, "Well I *have* gotten a couple of promotions since 2003, but how can you tell?" And her response was, "Because, you have gotten FAT!" and she laughed. I knew exactly why she said that – she wasn't being rude, she was being honest. Culturally, being overweight and having more than enough food to get fat with was a symbol of success and high status. So she was actually just complimenting me on my success!

And there you had it. I was successful. And, I was fat.

Not long after that, I began to have these bouts of a racing heartbeat, like I was having a panic attack or a minor heart attack, so I went to my doctor and got a full work-up. The results showed that I had high blood pressure, an elevated pulse rate, high triglycerides, my LDL/HDL ratio was high, and I weighed 187 pounds at a height of 5'7". My doc pointed out that when I had begun seeing him about 10 years prior, my charts showed my weight at 160. And that extra weight now was mostly around my midsection, which had increased substantially. He explained the things that were going on, and that he was going put me on blood pressure medication, and if it didn't improve, maybe something to slow my heart rate, and I said, WAIT. Give me some time to drop some weight, ok? I know I can do better.

Dr. Sunny's comments (and my own doctor's comments and physical reality check) hit me particularly hard. I kept asking myself, "How did this happen???"

You see, I had been fat when I was a kid. I was bullied because of it. And I wasn't particularly athletic (I was a band geek), which didn't help any. To top it off, I ended up being a late bloomer. While all my friends in 6th grade were hitting puberty and growing and changing physically, I didn't. In fact, by the time I started 7th grade at the junior high school, I was still the same chubby small-ish kid, while it seemed all my buddies were becoming young men. Fortunately, at that time, I started a newspaper route and depending on the weather either walked or rode my bike for a couple hours every day (my route had 156 houses spread around multiple neighborhoods). I credit this activity with helping jump-starting my move into puberty because not long after that, my body finally started to change.

Around that same time, I saw the movie *Rocky* with Sylvester Stallone. Wow! Those training workout scenes were impressive! Right then I knew what I had to do – I needed to get pumped up! And I did. I voraciously read books and magazines about lifting weights and bodybuilding, including Arnold Schwarzenegger (what an inspiration!) and began to hit the weight room at the local YMCA religiously. Within a couple of years I grew, matured, and built out a pretty decent physique. Needless to say, I gained a lot of confidence and respect in myself, the bullying stopped, and guys started asking ME how to work out and get in better shape!

That began a nearly life-long interest in fitness, health, and a brief stint doing some amateur bodybuilding. I lifted weights as a hobby throughout high school and college. After I graduated college, I competed in an amateur bodybuilding show, the 1987 Intermediate Mr. Illinois, and took 4th place in the lightweight class (I was fairly muscular and ripped, but not huge and massive).

When I went back to school to study a master's program, I got a job as a fitness instructor and trainer at a local health club. It was a fun gig, and I really enjoyed helping people learn how to work out, eat better, and get healthier. I remember working with clients who were in their 40s, sporting bellies and thinking to myself, *"man, I would NEVER let myself go like that. I will always keep myself in tip-top shape!"*

Fast-forward 25 years, and here I was, 49 years old, sporting a gut and being told by a nice Chinese doctor that I had gotten fat, and my physical showed I was borderline in need of medication to control my blood pressure and heart rate!!

The question now was, what do I do about it? Well, serendipity is a beautiful thing. Because at that time, JD Griffin, an old friend I used to work out with in high school had recently reached out to me. I was a medical editor and publisher, and he said he'd written a book on doing a body transformation after he found himself in his mid-40s and fat, and he wanted to pick my brain about publishing it. Long story short, I ended up serving as his book's editor, and even better, I told him I was going to do his transformation program with the goal of getting my health and my abs back for my 50th birthday.

I followed his program to a T and had amazing success. The book is called *"Get Fit, Lean, and Keep Your Day Job: A Transformation Guide for Any Body"* – I highly recommend reading it! GetFitLean really was leveraging a moderately low-carb diet to lose fat, and a specific high intensity workout plan to gain muscle. In 16 weeks I went from weighing nearly 190 pounds to my college weight of 150 pounds (in fact, I got down to 147 at one point). And I was sporting a nice deep 6-pack for my 50th birthday. Not to mention that my blood pressure normalized, my triglycerides were back to where they should be, and all my other health parameters were right where they should be.

The low-carb GetFitLean program really worked wonders, but it was low-carb, not keto. I found myself sometimes lacking energy and being a little brain-fogged because I was reducing my glucose levels, but not drastically enough to cause my body to produce ketones which would have provided plenty of energy.

Serendipity raised its hand again. One of my former coworkers from the health club I worked at way back in grad school reached out to me. He had seen my transformation pictures on Facebook, and saw me extolling the virtues of low-carb eating.

"What do you know about ketones and ketosis?" he asked. Now, I knew a little from what I heard of the Atkins diet, but I didn't really know that much. I knew it was hard to get into ketosis, and after some input from him and a little online research, I began to read about how being in ketosis provided a lot of potential health benefits. I wanted to know what he was doing, and he explained a company he was working with was about to launch an exogenous ketone supplement that you could drink, and get into ketosis in 60 minutes. I told him I had to try it. That supplement changed my life, and piqued my interest about ketosis.

I felt so good, both from a mental and also an energy standpoint, that I had to find out more about ketones and ketosis. Being a medical publisher, I delved into the National Library of Medicine's PubMed database of medical research, and found a lot of very interesting studies about the ketogenic diet, ketosis, and ketone bodies themselves. I began experimenting with ketogenic nutrition as well as low-carb variations, and supplementing with therapeutic ketones, and right now, in my mid-50s (I am 55 at the time of this writing) I look and feel fantastic, and I know other people could too. My passion for the last several years has been sharing this knowledge with others, and it is culminating in this book!

I hope I haven't lost your attention with this semi-novel, but I'm telling you this because **we all have a story, and we all have the opportunity to write and rewrite our story as life happens!** My point to all this is this:

I wasn't born in great shape, or a skilled athlete, or a nutrition expert. I have worked hard to become those things. I've been fat, and I've been fit, and I've been fat again, and now I'm even more fit! So, I know what it takes to make a decision to commit to changing your lifestyle to improve your health. I've helped many people get healthier, feel better, and look better, and I believe the information in this book will provide the framework for you to do the same!

Now, I met my amazing co-author, Dr. Lori Shemek, through JD Griffin, as he recommended I read her books "Fire Up Your Fat Burn," and "How to Fight FATflammation!" (PS: they are great books! You should also read them!) Dr. Lori and I both have a strong affinity for education, coaching, and helping people achieve their health, nutrition, fitness, and weight loss goals. Her empathy and desire to help others is so strong, and she really has a way about her that connects with people. As a result of a lot of conversations about ketones and ketogenic nutrition, we decided to collaborate on this book. Lori and I present to you, *The Ketogenic Key!*

- Steve Welch

INTRODUCTION

First of all, thank you for purchasing this book! We're so excited to be writing a definitive and simple guide to ketosis – where the "KEY" is ketosis, and the book covers multiple ways of achieving ketosis, such as the ketogenic diet and ketogenic therapies. Our goal with this book is to introduce you to the amazing state of ketosis, as well as the ketogenic lifestyle, and give you the "key" to unlock and fire up a high-performance way of living that will change your life. Ketosis is a state of optimal performance for the human body and brain, and we are going to show you how to achieve and maintain it!

In this book we will explore how to get into ketosis, describe the many ways it's beneficial to your health and well-being, walk you through the process of how to get into ketosis through diet, fasting, exercise, and supplementation, and give you guidance on foods and recipes that will help ensure that you can achieve ketosis and maintain a higher level of health, vitality, cognitive function, longevity and fitness than ever before.

We'll also dispel some common myths and misconceptions about ketosis. Behind this all, we will cite and describe the science and research supporting our statements and beliefs because as we write this book, there is an explosion of research, clinical trials, and scientific interest in ketosis, the ketogenic diet, and ketone supplementation.

The other thing we want you to know is that we're not just writing about the concepts in this book as a PhD researcher and a guy with an interest in nutrition. *We are actually experienced practitioners of ketogenic nutrition and lifestyle, including the ketogenic diet, intermittent fasting, exercise techniques, and using ketone supplements,* all of which have had a tremendous positive impact on our health, energy levels, mental and cognitive function, and overall well being. That's why we're so excited to share all of this with you – because <u>we know from personal experience that these techniques</u>

<u>work!</u> Read our bios to find out more about our personal experiences.

Ketosis is not new. It's really the natural state our bodies are meant to operate in if we were eating the way our ancestors ate. The ketogenic diet (keto) is not a "fad" diet. It has been used for medical purposes for ages. Although it was used as a treatment and cure for epilepsy and other medical conditions nearly a century ago, it got lost in the "drugs are more convenient" mindset starting around the 1940s and 50s. However, it is rapidly re-gaining respect in the medical community, and mainstream popularity. In recent years it has been "rediscovered" and touted as a weight loss and fitness miracle by celebrities like Halle Berry, Khloé Kardashian, and many others. Medical contributors like Dr. Josh Axe and Dr. Oz have talked about its health benefits on TV news shows – and we should know, because Dr. Shemek has appeared on TV on "The Doctors" program herself! Keto has been embraced by major pro athletes such as LeBron James in a number of sports. Team Sky, who won the 2018 Tour de France, were rumored (and later confirmed) to be using ketone supplements as part of their athletic performance toolkit, prompting more than a dozen teams to start using them in the 2019 Tour de France. And even more exciting, the ketogenic diet and ketogenic supplementation have become the subject of many clinical patient trials to test their potential to help medical conditions like diabetes and obesity, heart disease, depression and mood disorders, Alzheimer's disease and dementia, neurologic diseases, and even cancer.

Ketosis is highly regarded with very good reasons by such a broad range of medical professionals, researchers, athletes, celebrities, and fitness and health experts. As we mentioned before, it's not a fad. The fact is, ketosis is a natural state of being, and the ketogenic diet is a very natural way of eating. Keto (or something close to it) was probably the basic diet of our ancestors thousands of years ago. Did you know that you're born into a state of ketosis, and that mother's milk is one of the most ketogenic foods found in nature? Babies don't typically move away from a ketotic state until they stop breast-feeding and are given carbohydrate-filled baby foods, fruit juices, and processed flour and grain-based foods! Ketosis is natural and essential for your physical and neurological development as a baby. Sadly, many of the chronic conditions and diseases we develop as we age are a direct result of eating foods

Section 1: The Basics

that our bodies are not designed or meant to eat, and moving away from the kind of diet nature intended us to eat, which keeps us out of that magical state of ketosis for most of our lives!

Getting into ketosis and following a ketogenic nutrition regimen will move us back into the way of eating that feeds our bodies the right way, reduces inflammation, and trains our body to use fat for fuel instead of storing it on our bodies.

In addition, the keys to achieving a healthy state of ketosis include intermittent fasting, ketone supplementation, and exercise – and we'll discuss all of these things in the chapters that follow.

When Dr. Shemek wrote her first two books, *"Fire Up Your Fat Burn"* and *"How to Fight FATflammation"*, her goal was to help people improve their health by losing fat and reducing inflammation in their bodies. This book complements those two books perfectly, because ketosis, ketogenic eating, intermittent fasting, and ketone supplementation have been proven to both help people lose fat and quell insidious chronic low-level inflammation.

We know you'll enjoy getting started on this new lifestyle. Achieving ketosis is a powerful health tool. The keto diet, for example, is a pretty simple diet, but it takes a bit of getting used to. Ketone supplementation is a very new complementary strategy, and intermittent fasting has long been seen as "extreme" but is gaining widespread popularity and respect as a healthy way of eating. Starting anything new can be challenging. But ultimately once you achieve the state of ketosis, you'll feel so much better, both physically and mentally, that you'll be happy to avoid carbs, experiment with intermittent fasting, exercise more, and educate yourself about potential supplements. The Ketogenic Key is ready to help you unlock a better lifestyle!

Are YOU ready? Then let's get to it!

The Ketogenic Key
Section 1: The Basics

Chapter 1: What is Ketosis – And Why Should You Care?

You've probably heard people at work, at the gym, on TV – especially on the news or even celebrities themselves – talking about "keto" this and "keto" that – as well as the ketogenic diet and the recently available ketone supplements. We're going to talk a lot in this book about what we consider the Ketogenic Key: *getting into the state of ketosis* – and we'll be discussing the ketogenic diet at length in this book, but before we do that, let's take a step back and talk about what exactly "keto" means. Basically, "keto" is short for "ketogenic." Ketogenic means, "creating ketones" ("keto" for ketones, and "genic" for genesis, or creation). So a ketogenic diet is a diet that causes your body to create ketones.

Which begs the next question: what are ketones, and why should you care? Well, listen up, because this is the part that is going to change your life! Ketones are molecules that our body and brain use for energy, and that have numerous health benefits, which we will tell you all about. Now, when we have an elevated level of ketones in our body, that is what's called "ketosis," and the primary goal of this book is to lay out exactly how and why you would want to get into a state of ketosis – and how **(1) the ketogenic diet, (2) exogenous ketone supplements, (3) intermittent fasting, and (4) exercise** can all work separately or in tandem to help you achieve this excellent state of being: Ketosis! We believe that once you hear about all the things ketones and ketosis can do for you, you'll probably be willing to run through a brick wall to get them circulating in your body and brain! Although, there's a much simpler way.... Or ways! We'll touch on all of them in detail.

Ketone Bodies Explained

In this book, when we talk about ketones, we are talking about the 3 specific ketone bodies that are produced in the liver from fatty acids during periods of low carbohydrate or food consumption, fasting, starvation, or prolonged high intensity exercise. They are acetoacetate, acetone, and beta-hydroxybutyrate (BHB). As noted before, they are used by the body for energy, and are readily used by tissues all over the body, including the brain. BHB is present in the highest levels and is considered better for cell energy production and brain energy metabolism. This is important because the brain is a very energy-hungry organ, and we'll talk a lot about how ketones positively impact your brain from an energy and a cellular perspective.

Ketones (especially BHB) also serve as signaling molecules, sending messages to your body to regulate energy, metabolism, anti-inflammatory processes, and gene expression. In addition, recent research has shown that the ketone body acts as a ligand for key receptors in the body and activates processes that are similar to neurotransmitters and hormones. The receptors bind to other molecules that regulate the function of neurons that control our body's metabolic rate.

BHB is an incredibly useful, valuable, and hard-working molecule! It's no wonder people who achieve ketosis seem to enjoy so many health benefits.

So, next, let's talk about *ketosis.*

Ketosis Explained

Earlier we defined what ketogenic means. So what exactly does "ketosis" mean? Well for the purposes of this book, we define "ketosis" as a state of being where your body has a therapeutic level of ketones circulating in your bloodstream. Now, getting your body into a state of ketosis isn't magic. It is simply proven science and biology. Ketosis is a natural occurrence that happens when you don't feed your body carbohydrates and it exhausts its stores of glucose, or when you restrict your calorie intake significantly, and it is forced to look for energy elsewhere. Where does it look? Well, one place it looks for energy is fat – either your stored body fat or fat that you eat – which it can convert into ketone bodies to use for energy.

Chapter 1: What is Ketosis – And Why Should You Care?

You have possibly experienced very short-term ketosis when you've missed a couple of meals or have exhausted your body's supply of glucose because of rigorous or long-lasting endurance exercise. Even sleeping for long periods (without eating) can prompt your body's production of ketones! Whenever you exhaust your body's typical fuel supply of readily available glucose and glycogen, your body helps you out by raising its level of ketones, its alternative fuel source. However, most people eat enough sugar and carbs to keep their glucose levels relatively high all day and night – and thus keep ketosis from ever happening. You see, if you have any appreciable amount of glucose in your body, it senses that fuel is available and it won't produce ketones, and thus you won't go into a state of nutritional ketosis. But there are multiple ways to impact your body's glucose and glycogen levels, as well as boost your ketone levels. That's why, in this book, we delve into more than just the ketogenic diet as the way(s) to get your body into ketosis.

For the moment, let's talk about carbohydrates. Humans love sugar and carbs, no matter how bad they are for us, and our bodies happily and easily use them as fuel. And since our body is very efficient and smart, and wants to help us out if we ever have a reduction in available fuel, it takes any excess glucose and other calories that we eat and stores it as body fat for future use as energy. Stored fat translates into the not-so-funny belly fat that we never want.

Because carbohydrates so quickly and easily convert to glucose, the more you restrict your carbohydrate consumption, the more likely your body will have to produce ketones to fuel itself. It really has no other options. When we restrict the amount of carbohydrates that we eat, our body will still provide us with energy, but it must turn to another source. And that alternate source is fat, which has been so thoughtfully stored by our body for emergencies. The result is that your body goes into a state of *ketosis* and *ketogenesis*, where it's producing ketones from those fatty acids and glycerol, circulating them through the body and brain, and using them for energy.

So, to be very clear: **Ketosis is the natural process the body goes through when deprived or depleted of glucose and other sources of energy.**

Researchers have discovered much of what they know about ketosis from people who fast (do not eat for long periods of time), thereby depriving them of all sources of energy. After two days of fasting, the body will start to produce *ketones* as it breaks down the available protein and begins to use stored fat for fuel.

Obviously, achieving ketosis by following a ketogenic diet or by fasting would be healthier than starving yourself. Ketogenic eating should ideally become a lifestyle action that is driven by the goal to achieve and maintain ketosis and enjoy the benefits ketosis can have on your body and brain, rather than briefly trying a ketogenic diet as a quick weight-loss method.

One of the reasons ketosis is so beneficial is that ketones offer protection against some types of diseases, inflammation, and oxidative damage that can affect the body. Ketosis is an excellent way to maintain longevity, health, and strength for years, even decades!

This statement about longevity is not hyperbole, nor just our opinion. Emerging science and research continues to show how reducing carbohydrate consumption and being in ketosis can improve morbidity and mortality, as well as cell longevity and regeneration. In a study published August 29, 2017 in *the Lancet*, scientists concluded "A high carbohydrate intake was associated with an adverse impact on total mortality, whereas fats including saturated and unsaturated fatty acids were associated with lower risk of total mortality and stroke. We did not observe any detrimental effect of fat intakes on cardiovascular disease events."

A September 5, 2017 study found that a ketogenic high-fat, low-carb diet extended longevity and health span.

Another recent study showed that ketone bodies delayed senescence (programmed cell death) of cells in the vascular system, essentially keeping blood vessels and cells "younger."

So, as you can see, ketosis is a natural state of physical being with a host of benefits. In another section, we'll delve into the many diverse potential benefits of a ketogenic lifestyle!

A Clarification: Ketosis vs Diabetic Ketoacidosis

A frequent misconception that we hear from people, including some medical professionals and dieticians/nutritionists, is that ketones are bad for you. Why would they say this? Well, because some diabetics with uncontrolled blood sugar can develop a condition called "diabetic ketoacidosis" in which their blood sugar and ketones levels both get toxically high. It is extremely important to understand the fact that this dangerous condition (*diabetic ketoacidosis*) is NOT the same as being in a healthy and natural state of *ketosis*, and that ketones in and of themselves are actually a healthy and normal part of your body's metabolic process. We'll delve into this more in the section on common myths and misconceptions. But it's crucial right away to assure you that ketosis is nothing like ketoacidosis, but they are often confused with each other by people because they sound similar. In addition, many healthcare professionals associate ketones with something negative because the only thing they teach in medical school is that high levels of ketones might mean a patient has ketoacidosis.

The bottom line is that ketosis is healthy (babies are born in a state of ketosis and stay there as long as they consume mother's milk) and the ketogenic diet, fasting, and ketone supplementation can help achieve a healthy therapeutic state of ketosis, and are not causes of ketoacidosis.

Chapter 2:

The 4 Methods For Getting Into Ketosis and Staying There!

1.   **The Ketogenic Diet**
2.   **Intermittent Fasting**
3.   **Ketone Supplementation**
4.   **Exercise**

So, now that you know what our Ketogenic Key is (hint: ketosis!), and why ketosis is SO good for your body and brain, health, and longevity, let's discuss 4 ways that you can achieve and maintain ketosis. Now, all of these can work individually, although some make it easier to achieve ketosis on their own than others (*i.e.*, getting into ketosis with a ketogenic diet alone is easier than getting into ketosis with exercise alone). But when you combine 2 or more of these methods, you will find it MUCH easier to achieve – and maintain – a state of ketosis!

Getting Into Ketosis and Staying There

Method 1: The Ketogenic Diet

The ketogenic (keto) diet is a low- or zero-carbohydrate diet that differs from other low-carb diets in that it deliberately manipulates the ratios of carbs, fats, and protein in order to switch the body's primary source of fuel from glucose (sugar) to fats (which are used to generate ketone bodies by the liver). And that's exactly what it boils down to: when we go into a state of ketosis, we want our bodies making ketones (by way of fat breakdown) and using them for fuel.

When we eat a normal Western diet that is moderate to high in carbohydrates, our bodies get used to breaking down those carbohydrates into glucose and using that as an immediate, short-acting fuel. In fact, when we eat carbohydrates, they become the body's first-line or preferred source of fuel. Fats, which are also a potential source of fuel, are rarely or never used by our bodies if there are plenty of carbohydrates being consumed and making plenty of glucose hit our bloodstream. As a result, most people have plenty of fat on their bodies and fat in their diet that could be used as fuel, but they never are able to get their body to tap into and use that fat. On a Western diet, people eat too many carbohydrates, and almost always too many calories. That results in the extra calories being stored as fat, and our body keeps adding on the pounds as we continue this way of eating.

The only ways to reduce body fat when eating a "normal" Western high-carbohydrate diet are to consume fewer calories and exercise a lot in order to increase energy expenditure, so that our level of calories burned is more than our daily caloric intake. This is why most people fail to lose weight on conventional diet. It's very hard to out-exercise a bad (high carb) diet!

On the other hand, the ketogenic diet is very low in carbohydrates, which coaxes your body to use fat for fuel (energy). That means fat gets burned instead of being stored. As a result, weight loss and fat loss become much easier.

How does the keto diet get your body to use fat for fuel?

Normally your body easily and quickly uses carbohydrates for fuel. Carbs break down into glucose (sugar) and are a fast but short-lived source of energy. But when you reduce the amount of carbohydrates you're eating, your body doesn't have that easy quick fuel and must turn to its other fuel source, ketones. Your body makes ketones when it switches fuel sources and begins breaking down fat into ketones.

Therefore, the KEY of the ketogenic diet is to get your body into the state of "ketosis," where it has a healthy level of ketones circulating in your body, and it is using those ketones as fuel for your body and brain. In fact, ketones are a better, more efficient source of energy than glucose, because they generate approximately 38% more energy than glucose.

> *"An important takeaway is that we all have the ability to switch our metabolism from glucose to ketone utilization. And that switch has the potential to have profound health benefits for us, in addition to the positive changes in body composition."*

~Stephen Anton, **Associate Professor and Chief, Division of Clinical Research,** College of Medicine at the University of Florida

Why are ketones a superior fuel than glucose?

When you are following a ketogenic diet and get into the state of ketosis, you are fueling your body with exactly what it needs, while eliminating toxins and reducing the inflammatory aspects of a normal Western diet. The keto diet focuses on eating very few grams of carbohydrates and eating more fats, which the body converts into fuel to provide better energy; this in turn encourages fat usage and fat loss.

Chapter 2

What exactly is the problem with eating a lot of carbs, and why should you avoid them?

When you eat carbohydrates, they are very quickly converted into glucose (sugar) in your bloodstream. Now, glucose is a very easily used fuel for your body, but in large quantities in the bloodstream, it can be toxic. Therefore, our body uses the insulin to move glucose out of the blood stream. So, the quick conversion of carbohydrates that you eat, into glucose in your bloodstream, causes your body to release a spike of insulin, which is the hormone that takes glucose from your bloodstream and shuttles it to your cells to use as energy. Unfortunately, that creates a different problem. You see, insulin is also a hormone that signals your body to store extra calories as body fat. And when we eat a large amount of carbohydrates during a meal, only a small portion of those can be immediately used as energy. That means the rest will end up stored as fat. So, that in a nutshell is the issue with carbs. Carbs raise blood sugar, which causes as a spike in insulin, which then also results in the storage of fat. The insulin moves the glucose to your cells for energy – and any surplus glucose and other fat and protein calories that you've eaten will get stored as fat.

The Problem With Carbs: Fat Storage and Inflammation

Carbohydrates pose a two-pronged problem. First, people tend to eat far more carbs than their body needs for immediate energy, and carbs spike our blood glucose and initiate an insulin response, which signals the body to store those calories as fat. To add insult to injury, insulin is also a very inflammatory hormone, so its repeated circulation every time we eat a high-carb meal and snack on carbs, also causes inflammation in our bodies.

And of course, as long as there are carbs and glucose from our diet readily available to use for fuel, our body will never look for an alternative energy source. Therefore, the more carbs you consume in your daily diet, the less likely that fat is being burned for energy. Instead, the spike in glucose and the subsequent insulin spike caused by eating those carbohydrates will result in more fat storage, inflammation, and the creation of free radicals and reactive oxygen species (ROS), which are very harmful to your body on a cellular level.

This is why ketosis is such a powerful state of physical being. Basically, being in ketosis allows your body to change the way it uses energy from glucose to fat (*i.e.,* ketones) – and ketones are a more efficient, cleaner energy source than glucose. Ketones have even been shown in clinical studies to inhibit inflammation, rather then promote it the way insulin does. So in so many ways, being in ketosis and getting your body to use ketones as fuel, has a domino effect of excellent health benefits!

Another important thing to understand is that being in ketosis helps the body fuel itself on less food. By being in ketosis, you "train" your body to utilize fats as the main source of energy instead of carbs, because there are very few carbohydrates eaten to use as fuel. Through a process called "ketogenesis," the liver breaks down those fats and creates ketones, which enables the body to use the fat as energy. There's a misconception that the ketogenic diet is a starvation diet, and that's just not true. During a keto diet, we don't starve ourselves of calories – on keto you can eat a lot of rich and satiating, fatty foods like avocado, cheese, eggs, bacon, butter and more. The only starvation that occurs during a keto diet, is that we starve the body of carbohydrates, which only means it MUST turn to fat as fuel! This makes weight loss easy and natural.

The Hybrid Car Analogy

One way to look at it is to think of your body as a hybrid car. It can run on two fuels: carbohydrates (glucose and sugar), or fats (ketones). Carbs burn very quickly and don't last, and like gasoline, they cause a dirty "exhaust" at the cellular level from the inflammation, free radicals, and reactive oxygen species, which damage your cells and blood vessels. Ketones, on the other hand, are like the electric portion of the hybrid: they burn long, steady, and clean! And because they generate more energy than glucose, ketones are actually more biologically economical than carbs and glucose.

Ketosis = Healing

In addition to weight loss, the ketogenic diet is known as the "healing" diet. Reducing carb and sugar intake has been proven to help prevent, manage, and in some case even reverse the negative effects of diseases such as heart disease, high blood pressure, high triglycerides, cancers, epilepsy, and many symptoms of aging. In fact, research shows that people with different types of cognitive issues, from Parkinson's disease to epilepsy, can improve brain function tremendously by switching from glucose to ketones for brain energy metabolism.

We'll get into more detail about the numerous benefits of ketones, ketosis, and the ketogenic diet in the next few chapters. But suffice to say that keto can be healing and can result in numerous improvements in your health quality!

Ketogenic Diet vs. Other Diets

Many people confuse the ketogenic diet with low carb diets or paleo diets. There are so many different diets in the news, and there is a lot of misinformation about the ketogenic vs other diets. So, there are considerable differences of which you should be aware. Let's address these other diets, just so we are clear on what we mean when we talk about keto, as well as make sure you understand the differences between keto and other diets.

Keto vs. Low-Carb

A low-carb diet can be anything it wants to be, as long as it is low in carbohydrates. However, the issue with saying a diet is "low carb" is that "low" is rarely defined or quantified. How low is low? Often times, with a "low-carb" diet, people simply make random food choices that curb their carb intake arbitrarily. If there is no real targeted number, they might still be consuming too many carbs to achieve their health or fat loss goals. In general, a commonly used range for low-carb is between 75-150 grams of carbs daily, although some experts (and we agree) recommend eating less than 100 grams daily for a most effective low-carb regimen.

Although a low-carb diet is a good start, and may help people improve their health to a degree and achieve some success in weight-loss, what the low-carb diet lacks is that all-critical ketogenic state that turns fat into fuel and provides your body with a new and effective source of energy: ketones. Without this, a low-carb diet can leave you feeling very hungry and tired. You see, cutting carbs is effective, but if you don't cut carbs enough to achieve ketosis, you are not consuming enough carbohydrates to meet your energy needs, and your body will turn to cannibalizing muscle tissue for energy, which is NOT what we want it to do.

The ketogenic diet has a specific ratio of carbs to fats to protein, and the carbs must be low enough to make your body turn to ketogenesis to fuel itself. This manipulation is critical, and it's why a simple low carb diet won't work as well, if at all, for getting you into ketosis. As mentioned previously, for a ketogenic diet to achieve nutritional ketosis, it should consist of 70-80% fats, 20-25% protein, and 10% or less carbs (ideally 5% or less). Anything above that amount of carbs, or eating too much protein, will not induce ketosis. And that's the difference. Low-carb does not mean ketogenic.

Keto vs. Paleo

The paleo diet is also a low-ish carb-type diet, but not specifically ketogenic. It is based on the assumption that eating the way our hunter-gatherer Paleolithic cavemen ancestors did (*i.e.*, meat, vegetables, nuts/seeds and fruit, and no processed flours, sugars or grains) is a healthy way of eating. And although that may very well be true, it's not a diet that will help you achieve ketosis.

The paleo diet advocates removing processed grains and processed foods, which is a good thing for anyone, but the fruit, starchy vegetables and other foods with carbs will provide too many grams of carbohydrates and prevent getting into ketosis. So it's important to understand that while paleo may have health benefits, it is not ketogenic by design.

Keto vs. Whole30

The Whole30 diet means that you eliminate foods that are processed and can cause inflammation, and only eat whole, intact, unprocessed foods for 30 days. Like Paleo, this is not a bad thing, and we encourage anyone to cut processed foods from their diet, and encourage eating whole, intact foods. However, the Whole30 diet is not necessarily low carb, and will not result in achieving ketosis. In addition, some people find it too restrictive and don't stay on it past the initial 30 days. Although the program encourages long-term adherence, many people think of it as a temporary diet to encourage changing your eating habits. Now, we have heard of people who have used Whole30 to help them change how they eat and think of food, and then transitioned to a ketogenic diet once they felt "in control" of their nutrition and eating. If that works for them, we applaud it!

Dirty Keto vs. Clean Keto

Ketosis changes lives. However, it is very important to be aware of big business's promotion of what we call "dirty keto" as the latest keto hack. Dirty keto is basically eating processed foods or fast food menu items that technically fit the macros of the keto diet (the correct amount of fat and protein and low in carbs). Whereas we are promoting clean eating with real, whole, unprocessed foods as a part of the keto diet, dirty keto is taking advantage of people's desire and need for convenience by way of eating packaged, fast, or processed foods.

Well, we all know it was bound to happen. As more and more people are interested in "going keto," food manufacturers want to capitalize on consumer desire for convenient, pre-packaged foods that are very low in carbohydrates and higher in fat. Those food manufacturers see the potential dollar signs of cashing in on the popularity of keto! So they are offering products that technically meet the definition of keto because of their macros, but may not be in the best interest of your health. And in today's culture of immediate gratification, there will be plenty of people who only want to adhere to the letter of the keto law, not the spirit, so those food manufacturers are salivating with every unhealthy keto bar they sell. Be careful. When you think of *dirty keto,* think inflammation and processed foods.

Why is dirty keto unhealthy? Here is the problem. Different types of proteins and fats have a different effect upon the body. Technically, you could drink diet sodas, have sticks of processed margarine with a side of trans-fat loaded pork rinds and it could be called "keto" because it's low carbs and high in fat, and yes, you could potentially make it into ketosis – but at a potentially serious cost to your body and health. These companies could (and most likely will) put cheap highly processed protein and fats into their keto bar or keto cookies, such as soy protein isolate, which may have a negative impact on your body at the cellular level. So what is happening, unfortunately, is the unhealthy trend of dirty keto.

We get it. It's so tempting to think that you can breeze through the fast food joints and maintain ketosis. We also understand that this can be a huge timesaver if you are not having to meal plan and prepare real food – you're eating tasty food and yet keeping your carbs low. Granted, doing this once in a while is fine, such as when traveling or when your schedule will not permit you to prepare and eat real foods. Just make sure it's a rare occurrence and not a common one. Remember, the *quality* of the food you eat has a powerful effect upon cellular health, hormones, sleep, weight and overall health outcomes. But the real issue with dirty keto, or eating processed and unhealthy foods to try to achieve ketosis, is the lack of high food quality, the drop in micronutrients, and the fact that you are putting unhealthy foods into your body instead of healthy ones.

Dirty keto may fit the bill as a rare, temporary fix, or a meal of convenience. Just don't make a habit of it or build your long-term meal plans around it. If you are going to do some dirty keto meals here and there, ensure you get the necessary vitamins, minerals, fiber, and other nutrients from other high-quality foods to protect your overall health.

Examples of dirty keto (with some of the potential negative aspects parenthetically listed):

- Diet Soda (remember, artificial sweeteners can still raise your insulin levels, and diet soda has been shown to be highly inflammatory)
- Bunless Fast Food Burger with Cheese and Bacon (often times fast food meat quality is very low and lacking in nutrients, and fast food cheese is typically not real cheese; it's low quality processed cheese-like food)
- Fast Food Egg and Sausage Sandwich Guts (*i.e.,* no bread) – (typically low quality meats and egg substitutes or reconstituted dried egg powder)
- Pork Rinds (often sugar added and often processed with the lowest quality inflammatory vegetable oils, and may contain trans-fats)
- Beef Jerky (see above; often there is sugar added, and a lot of unhealthy preservatives to maintain shelf life)
- American Cheese or Cheese Foods (these are not "real" cheese)
- Protein Bars (often loaded with sugars or processed texturizers and preservatives)
- Sugar-Free Snacks (typically sugar is replaced by artificial sweeteners or sugar alcohols)
- Pre-packaged Protein Shakes (can have hidden sugars or low quality protein and loads of processed additives)
- Keto Bombs (made with poor quality fats and artificial sweeteners). Keto bombs made with quality coconut oil and grass-fed butter, natural pure cacao and peanut butter are ok though.
- Cheez Whiz (if it's spelled this way, it's not real cheese and basically a Frankenfood)
- Pre-Cooked Bacon (often with sugar or preservatives added)
- Keto Chips
- Milk Coffees (milk often contains added lactose, which is a type of sugar)
- Beef Sticks (see Jerky above)

The Bottom Line: keep your standards high with your keto food choices and focus on eating real, whole foods whenever possible. If it comes in a box or a package, it's probably processed to some degree.

Why Is the Ketogenic Diet So Effective and Healthy? The "Key" is Ketosis!

There are many reasons the ketogenic diet has such a profound impact on health. Achieving and maintaining a state of ketosis helps improve your overall physical and mental well being, in addition to helping you lose weight. You have more energy during the day, and you feel satiated and that desire for food disappears, thereby reducing the cravings for unhealthy snacks. In essence, you are eating less, but eating better. That's what makes the keto diet so unique and successful.

The ketogenic diet is not magic pill made up by some gurus. Countless research studies, case series, and anecdotal testimonials back the effectiveness of this diet. It is a scientifically proven method that balances your body's fat and protein intake, while reducing your carbohydrate intake, to help achieve optimal health and weight loss.

By using fat instead of glucose as your primary source of energy, the keto diet induces the state of **ketosis**, which is achieved when your body stops receiving carbohydrates to turn into glucose. The fewer carbohydrates you consume, the more you force your body to burn fat for energy instead of storing it.

This is why it is possible to lose weight so quickly when you're in ketosis from a ketogenic diet. You count carbohydrates instead of calories. Using fats as an energy source is what ketosis is all about. It is the natural metabolic state that helped our hunter-gatherer ancestors survive and thrive.

They feasted on low-carb foods when they could, and fasted when food was scarce. Fat was stored and converted into energy during the scarce times. The state of ketosis is a natural human state, and that makes the ketogenic diet so powerful and successful. In addition to all the physical benefits of ketosis, most people simply enjoy the way that being in ketosis makes them feel: better and more energetic.

Weight loss results on the keto diet differ among individuals, depending on their specific body composition. But weight loss has been the consistent result of people who've been on the keto diet.

Backed by Research

In addition to anecdotal evidence, more and more research is showing the impressive difference the ketogenic diet can make. Here are a couple of examples:

A 2017 study divided Crossfit training subjects into two groups, with both groups following the physical training, but only one group combined the ketogenic diet with the training. The results showed that those on the keto diet decreased their fat mass and weight far more than the other group.

The keto diet group showed an average of 3.5 kilo weight loss, 2.6 percent of body fat, and 2.83 kilos in fat mass, while the other group lost no weight, body fat or fat mass. Both groups showed similar athletic performance ability.

A 2012 study divided overweight children and adolescents into two groups; one was put on a keto diet, the other on a low-calorie diet. As in other keto studies, the children on the keto diet decreased their weight, fat mass, and lowered their insulin levels considerably more than the low-calorie group.

Besides more rapid weight loss, a decided advantage of the keto diet over a low-calorie diet is that people actually stick to the keto diet. A low-calorie diet will help you lose weight, but you may be constantly feeling hungry and deprived – the main reason most diets fail. Hunger and deprivation are not a part of the ketogenic lifestyle.

So in summary, there are many reasons to consider following a ketogenic diet. Getting into ketosis is not easy, but it's worth it. We'll talk more about the diet later in this book, but next we want to go over another method of achieving ketosis.

Getting Into Ketosis and Staying There

Method 2: Intermittent Fasting

Have you ever been in such a hurry that you skipped breakfast or you were too tired to eat dinner? If so, you were unwittingly utilizing the tool of **intermittent fasting**. Intermittent fasting means you only eat within a certain time window, and don't eat (fast) for the remaining period(s) of time.

Intermittent fasting works effectively because it is this cycling of feasting (feeding) and famine (fasting) that mimics the eating habits of our ancestors, and restores your body to a more natural state that allows a whole host of biochemical benefits to occur.

Digesting food takes hours and requires many complex bodily functions. When your body is not occupied with processing food, the beneficial functions of cellular repair, regeneration, and restoration can occur instead. This is why fasting is both healthy, and in many ways necessary, for optimal body function and health.

With a traditional Western diet, we have all been told that we need to eat three square meals a day plus snacks; this has been ingrained into our eating behavior from morning to night. We are surrounded by food 24 hours a day, and that is the crux of the problem. Research shows that your body cannot run optimally when there's a continuous supply of food and calories coming in that require your body to process them.

When you eat a typical high-carb Western diet throughout the day and never skip a meal, your body adapts to burning sugar (glucose) as its primary fuel, which stops your body from utilizing and burning stored fat. All those meals and snacks spike your blood sugar and elicit an insulin response to mobilize that sugar out of your blood stream and into your cells, either to burn for energy or to store as fat. As a result, you start becoming progressively more insulin-resistant, start gaining weight, and most efforts to lose weight may be met with frustration because of this vicious cycle.

Chapter 2

The Ketogenic Key has built-in success for most everyone who follows it – a true key to optimizing health and life. One key is of course, carbohydrate restriction via the ketogenic diet. And another of these keys is a complementary way of eating, that when combined with the ketogenic diet, produces an even more powerful effect – and this is called ***intermittent fasting.***

Because of the health and physiological benefits it produces, we believe everyone should practice some form of intermittent fasting. Ditching your "3 square meals" a day and continuous snacking will help your health in numerous ways, especially if you're battling diabetes, obesity and inflammation.

Intermittent fasting is quite well documented in science as well as history as an effective dietary strategy with many health and anti-aging benefits. Many cultures, religions, and philosophical followers have practiced it for thousands of years, for good reason. It is the way our bodies were meant to operate, because food was not available 24-7, 365 days per year!

What Is Intermittent Fasting, And What Does It Do?

In a nutshell, intermittent fasting is simply **eating within a specified window of time, and then abstaining from food and caloric beverages for periods of time without eating anything at all**. By extending the periods between your meals, your glucose and insulin levels will lower, which gives the body a chance to do what it does naturally to optimize health: tap into stored body fat for fuel, raise growth hormone levels, and stimulate multiple cellular and metabolic processes that are beneficial to us, that only happen when we are NOT eating. These periods without food allow your body to go through a process called *autophagy,* which is the process in which your body cleans out cellular debris and renews itself at a cellular level. Autophagy has also been shown to help reboot our immune system and improve its function.

"All The Magic Happens When We Don't Eat"

Both intermittent fasting and the ketogenic diet on their own are powerful. And because we want you to be successful with your efforts to improve your health, weight, brainpower, energy and much more, and to maximize your results, we suggest you try combining the ketogenic diet along with intermittent fasting for a few days a week.

Intermittent Fasting Benefits

From fasting for just a few hours each day to skipping meals for two days each week, intermittent fasting not only fuels weight loss, but protects your brain and heart, too. But fasting can be a little confusing, given all of the different types. We will break it down for you, including the best fasting plan for beginners, and the differences between 16/8 Fasting, Alternate-Day Fasting, and The Warrior Diet or the 5:2 Fast. But before we get into what intermittent fasting is all about, let us refresh your memory on the plethora of benefits with the keto diet.

Remember all of those keto diet benefits mentioned in the previous chapters? Weight loss, disease prevention, resolving insulin resistance, optimizing your mitochondrial function, and preventing cellular damage from occurring, to name a few. These and other benefits can be profoundly improved with the addition of a bit of intermittent fasting.

Intermittent fasting is not just a beneficial way of eating to optimize health and weight; it also makes life much easier. When fasting, you no longer have to be bogged down with the time spent preparing food, buying food or thinking about food – a huge time-saver. Another excellent gain is financial. You will love how much money you save each week when you skip a few meals as part of your intermittent fasting protocol!

But the big news is all of the health benefits created by this incredibly simple eating strategy. Just check out the list below!

Intermittent Fasting Alone Improves:

- Increased fat oxidation, which speeds up your fat loss throughout the day—even while you are at rest.
- Disease protection/prevention

- Improves immune function
- Lowers blood pressure
- Supports prevention or reversal of type 2 diabetes
- Raises insulin sensitivity
- Promotes leptin sensitivity
- Reduces triglycerides
- Lowers insulin
- Normalizes ghrelin (the hunger hormone)
- Reduces heart disease
- Reduce "bad" or oxidized LDL cholesterol
- Reduces cancer risk
- Reduces inflammation
- Increases longevity
- Increases mitochondrial health
- Promotes longevity of cells
- Increases and protects neurological health
- Fights hunger (yes!) and sugar cravings
- Stimulates autophagy (cellular debris cleanup)
- Increases human growth hormone (HGH) levels

Different Types of Intermittent Fasting

Despite what most believe, there is more than one type of intermittent fasting. **Time Restricted Eating,** also called **time-restricted feeding,** is a form of intermittent fasting that simply means you are eating during a certain set of hours each day. Intermittent fasting is eating *intermittently* such as every other day, every 12 hours, etc., and *fasting* the rest of the time (with no snacking).

Here are the most popular forms of intermittent fasting:

16/8 Protocol

This is the most popular protocol. You eat all of your daily calories within a shortened period — typically 6 to 8 hours — and fast for the remaining 14 to 16 hours. You can do this every day, or a few times a week.

Examples: You can adjust this window to make it work in your life:

- **If you start eating at:** 7:00 am, stop eating and start fasting at 3:00 pm
- **If you start eating at:** 11:00 am, stop eating and start fasting at 7:00 pm
- **If you start eating at:** 2:00 pm, stop eating and start fasting at 10:00 pm
- **If you start eating at:** 6:00 pm, stop eating and start fasting at 2:00 am.

24-Hour Fast

You restrict all food for 24 hours, once or twice a week. **Skipping two meals one day or one meal a day, where you are taking 24 hours off from eating.** For example, eating on a normal schedule: finishing a typical dinner at 8:00 pm, and then not eating again until 8:00 pm the following day. So you would eat your normal meals per day, and then occasionally pick a day to skip breakfast and lunch the next day.

Or eat a normal breakfast and then not eat again until breakfast the next day. Whichever meal you choose to eat, simply don't eat again until that same meal the next day.

Two examples: skipping breakfast and lunch 1 day of the week, and then another where you skip lunch and dinner one day, 2 days in a week.

5:2 Method

This method allows you to eat normally 5 days a week. The other 2 days are your "fasting" days, although you do still eat a little bit, keeping food intake between 500 and 600 calories. There is some debate as to whether this is true fasting, due to the allowance of a small amount of food during the 2 days.

The Warrior Diet

This form of intermittent fasting replicates the way ancient warriors ate. They consumed little (such as nuts or berries) or nothing during the day until the evening when they would eat their hunt. This is how we evolved genetically and physiologically. Basically this is fasting dinner-to-dinner, or under-eating for 20 hours and then eating a lot in a 4-hour window. Similar to the 5:2 method, there is some debate whether this is true fasting, due to the allowance of a small amount of food during the day.

One Meal A Day (OMAD)

This fasting protocol allows you to eat one meal a day and you choose what you wish to eat. The one meal a day diet utilizes a type of intermittent fasting referred also as 23:1, meaning a person spends 23 hours of the day fasting, leaving just 1 hour a day to eat, drink and consume calories. It is recommended that you select the same meal every day so that you are going 23 hours from one meal to the next. In other words, don't do dinner one day, and then breakfast the next, since that's only going to be 12 hours. Eat only dinner or lunch or breakfast consistently. This is one of the easiest and most common fasting protocols because it's so simple.

36 Hour Fasting

A 36-hour fast means that you fast one entire day. You finish dinner on day 1 at 7:00 pm for instance, and you would skip all meals on day 2, and not eat again until breakfast at 7:00 am on day 3, which puts you at 36 hours without eating.

48+ Hour Fasts

Longer fasting periods over 24 hours are generally done less frequently because they are considered more extreme and should be done by experienced people who've fasted before and/or are doing it with medical supervision. Only you can determine if these longer types of intermittent fasts are right for you. It is crucial to work closely with a physician to monitor yourself if you have health conditions such as diabetes or if you are obese.

Water Fast

Water fasting is a method of fasting where you do not consume anything besides water between 24 to 72 hours. It is linked with a lower risk of chronic diseases and much increased autophagy but also comes with concerns about health for people who have pre-existing medical conditions or who are not accustomed to fasting for longer periods of time.

Dry Fasting

Dry fasting is an extreme form of fasting that is done without any food or water. A soft dry fast includes showering and brushing teeth while an absolute dry fast (or black fast) is done without contact to any water. We only mention this as information only, and do not recommend black fasting. If you decide to try it, we recommend you consult your physician before embarking on this type of intermittent fasting.

The Intermittent Fasting Blueprint

Intermittent fasting is the process of cycling in and out of periods of eating and not eating.

The Fasting Window

There are 3 steps to the Fasting Window:

Step 1: Eat dinner the previous night at about 7:00 – 8:00 PM. Eating a meal with plenty of protein, fiber, and healthy fats is recommended to help minimize hunger the next day. That said, don't over-eat or gorge yourself with extra calories, or you may defeat the purpose of fasting in the first place. Eat a normal portioned meal.

Step 2: Fast throughout the night, and when you wake up in the morning, you should be in mild ketosis already. After you awaken, drink a glass of water (12 oz) with a pinch of sea salt. This will balance your electrolytes and reduce the stress of fasting. You can also have some black coffee or tea without dairy. We highly recommend green tea or a dark roast coffee to help support autophagy (cellular detox) and other health benefits. Don't drink any more than 2-3 cups of caffeinated coffee/tea. Some people recommend using a decaffeinated version so that you don't get jitters. Continue to drink more water during the fasting window.

Step 3: If you can, try to do some exercise while fasting to boost the benefits such as autophagy. Walking is particularly beneficial on an empty stomach. This low intensity aerobic activity will promote ketosis because you'll burn off remaining glucose stores, and help your body utilize fatty acids for energy.

The Feeding Window

Feeding, ah yes! Breaking a fast is a lesson in the true appreciation of food. When you eat, your body spends literally hours metabolizing food.

Let's assume your last meal was at 7:00 pm and you choose to fast until 11:00 am – a 16 hour fast. To break the fast, always choose a normal or slightly smaller meal consisting of healthy fats and/or protein. This will not put too much stress on the body and keep insulin and blood sugar balanced – eating a big meal with lots of carbs will spike your blood sugar and elicit an insulin spike, which is what we are trying to avoid in the first place! Stick to the Ketogenic Key Food List and eat as much as you feel comfortable with bearing in mind the carbohydrate and calorie count of foods.

Once we get over the idea that we need to eat every 3 or 4 hours, adapting to this schedule of eating easily overshadows any other diet or routine. Just do what you normally do and shorten the window of time when you eat, and lengthen the window of time when you don't eat.

As you can see, intermittent fasting is very easy, and becomes a superpower when combined with the ketogenic diet. In fact, following a keto diet makes intermittent fasting even easier, because eating a high-fat meal satiates your hunger for a longer period of time, making it a snap to skip meals during the IF day(s)!

Foods That Will Break Your Fast ("Red Light" Foods)

There are drinks or liquids that many people think are "safe" to have while fasting and in fact, stop the beneficial fasting process (we call these "red light" foods because they put a STOP to the benefits of fasting). Some seemingly insignificant foods promote an uptick in insulin. Even artificial sweeteners break a fast as the **artificial sweeteners can stimulate an insulin response.**

In general, **when fasting it is best not to consume calories of any kind, in order to stay in a fasted state.** This means sticking to liquids only, such as water, black coffee and unsweetened tea. Adding salt to your water can be beneficial as it will help you replenish your electrolytes and will not break your fast.

A couple of the major goals of fasting are to keep blood glucose levels down, and avoid increasing insulin secretion. By keeping the following foods out of your fasting window, you can be assured of receiving the top health benefits from fasting. Please note that some of these such as coconut oil and MCT oil are somewhat controversial. Some experts say such oils won't break your fast because they do not cause an insulin response, while others say they will, because they contain calories. The bottom line is to keep it simple and when in doubt, stick with pure liquids like black coffee, tea, and water.

Red Light Foods:

All dairy (whole cream, half and half, milk as well as cheese, sour cream etc.)
Stevia sweetener
Truvia sweetener

All artificial sweeteners (artificial sweeteners can trigger an insulin response)
Herbal teas with dried fruit
Nut milks
Coconut oil
MCT oil
MCT powder
Collagen powder

"Fat" coffee (coffee with butter, cream and coconut or MCT oil)
Bone broth
Branch chain amino acids (BCAAs)
Apple cider vinegar
Lemon juice
Butter
Whole foods

Foods That Are Safe During a Fast (Green Light)

Water
Sparking water (unsweetened)
Coffee
Tea – green, black, white, herbal – unsweetened of course!

Supplements

Some people recommend using supplements during fasting, and we would recommend that you do supplement with electrolytes and minerals – just be careful not to consume supplements that contain calories and potentially elicit that insulin response!

How To Use Intermittent Fasting With The Ketogenic Diet

Despite intermittent fasting's plethora of benefits, it can be a tough challenge the first week or two for some. However, for those of you following the Ketogenic Key guidelines, you will be fat adapted, or already well on your way to being fat-adapted.

If you have never fasted, it is important to do it simply and easily. For example, you can choose to delay breakfast an hour every day for 3 days, eventually eating your first meal as lunch. This means you will have an 8-hour eating window with two meals a day. Ultimately, your goal is to go at least 12 hours without eating or ingesting liquid calories. Conversely, you can do this with dinner – skipping dinner and eating breakfast and lunch only.

Assuming you do not eat breakfast, *it can take a good week to two weeks to stop thinking about breakfast.* Hunger feelings will occur – it's okay to be hungry, so try to distract yourself until lunchtime.

Having said this, it is very important to pay attention to bodily cues; be mindful. If you are doing intermittent fasting, and after the first few weeks it does not feel like a good fit for you, then it may not be after all. It's not for everyone.

What Is the Easiest Way to Begin Intermittent Fasting?

While intermittent fasting has many variations, the easiest way is to skip breakfast and make lunch your first meal—then, get all the calories you need in your lunch and dinner. The goal is not to starve yourself; it's to split your day into longer "fasting" periods and shorter "feeding" periods. This helps stimulate your body to simultaneously build muscle and burn fat. You are essentially training your body to burn fat for fuel and optimize your health.

The reason many people skip breakfast to establish their fasting window is because they've already been fasting when they wake up! Sleeping and not eating during the night is a natural fasting period, and if you add to the hours without food by not eating anything until lunch, you are increasing the benefits in a very simple and easy way. Research shows the longer you fast, the more benefits you accrue. Our bodies are very adaptable – you can "train" your appetite hormones to adjust quickly or slowly, depending upon which you choose.

Avoiding Common Fasting Mistakes

To make sure you'll gain both the fat burning, growth hormone boosting, and health-enhancing benefits of fasting, try to avoid these common mistakes:

- Fasting causes you too much stress
- Too much coffee
- Artificial sweeteners
- Food supplements while fasting (excluding minerals)
- Not fasting long enough
- Restricting calories too much
- Branched chain amino acids

Why do we mention stress? Because there's the concern of becoming too dogmatic and strict with fasting. You don't have to be perfect, so relax about it. Ensure that the combination of the ketogenic diet and intermittent fasting is not stressful for you. Levels of the stress hormone cortisol rise during tension-filled times. This can increase hunger, cravings, insulin levels, and weight, the exact opposite of what you ideally desire.

Fasting is an excellent way to achieve better health and weight loss and most importantly, for cellular health such as autophagy. Limiting yourself to unsweetened coffee, tea, and water, as well as salt in water will optimize your health and weight.

Always keep it simple and the results will follow. And if you'd rather not fast every day, or if you prefer doing shorter fasts (of 12-14 hours, for example), that's perfectly okay too – it's a very flexible strategy, and you shouldn't be apprehensive to experiment with it to see what works best for you. Heck, that's what we did!

Getting Into Ketosis and Staying There

Method 3: Ketone Supplementation – Achieving, Boosting, and Maintaining Ketosis with Exogenous Ketones

We'll spend the majority of this book describing how and why ketones are good for you, and how to get into a state of ketosis through your dietary choices, fasting protocols, and exercise. But we know that it may not be easy, or 100% permanent.

The reality is, many of you will try the ketogenic diet and/or intermittent fasting, but you may only do it for a limited period of time. Or you may find it difficult to adhere to such a strict diet every day, every meal. On top of that, ketosis can be a delicate state – once your body is in ketosis, it doesn't take much to knock it out of ketosis. If you slip up and accidentally (or even intentionally!) eat something with a bunch of carbs, you can knock your body out of ketosis and it can take days – or even weeks – to get back into a therapeutic state of nutritional ketosis. On top of that, some people can follow a very strict diet and only get their blood ketone levels into a slightly elevated level.

So, what if there was something you could just drink, that would put you in ketosis in an hour, and significantly boost the level of ketones circulating in your body? Well there is, and they're called *Exogenous Ketone Supplements.* There are several different types of ketone supplements, which we'll discuss in this chapter. First are ketone esters, second are racemic ketone salts, and third are MCT (medium-chain triglyceride) powders and oils.

The Origins of Ketone Supplementation

Years ago, the Department of Defense actually commissioned researchers to try to develop a ketone supplement that would minimize seizures that occur in Navy divers who are using high-oxygen rebreathers (breathing a high level of oxygen under pressure at deep depths can cause oxygen toxicity seizures). As we've mentioned previously, the ketogenic diet was used decades ago as treatment of epilepsy, and has made a comeback with increasingly common drug-resistant cases of epilepsy. DARPA and the Navy knew that there might be a way to develop an ingestible dose of ketones that would mitigate those oxygen toxicity seizures in divers. So researchers created a supplement and tested it. Interestingly, as the story goes, the side effects reported by the subjects included higher energy levels, less need for sleep, appetite suppression, mental clarity, and laser-like focus. That led to a high level of interest in creating a supplement for general soldiers, athletes, and other people who wanted to experience or benefit from these ketones.

Ketone Esters

The researchers knew they were onto something. However, synthesizing ketones into a supplement that humans can stomach was difficult, and it was expensive. Researchers at Oxford University successfully developed a ketone monoester. Early research showed the monoester was quite potent and worked well – in fact, a study on elite rowers showed that using the ketone monoester supplement resulted in improved performance, and several of the subjects attained personal bests. In addition, the researchers knew all of the benefits that ketones could have on energy, fat mobilization, cognitive improvement and more, including potential medical therapeutic interventions. However, making it widely available proved challenging because it was expensive to produce, and early taste testers claim it tasted absolutely disgusting. Although that didn't keep it from getting into the hands of those who wanted it.

Initially, these expensive and difficult to attain supplements were really only used by the "elite" who were in the know. It seemed that the only people who had access to ketone ester supplements were the military, scientific and medical researchers, and elite athletes who had a connection to someone who could provide them, as well as the money to afford them. For the past few years, Tour de France teams have been using ketone esters as their "secret weapon" to fuel and recover from the grueling pace of the Tour. It is rumored that Team Sky, who won the Tour in 2018, was using a monoester supplement as its secret (well, now not-so-secret) weapon, which lead to at least 13 teams rumored to be using them in the 2019 race.

More recently, at least 2 ketone monoester products have been released to the public. These ketone esters elevate blood ketone levels rapidly and significantly. Many athletes use them for events. In addition, due to their high potency, ketone esters are being studied for numerous health benefits in various clinical trials. Although many people still consider them to be too expensive for daily use by the average person, it's likely that with time, development costs will come down, and an affordable daily ketone monoester supplement will be a reality.

Ketone Salts

Looking for an alternative to expensive ketones monoesters, and a simpler way to product them, researchers developed supplements wherein ketones are bound to various mineral molecules such as sodium, calcium, potassium, and magnesium. Thus, ketone salt supplements have been brought to market. Although they are not as potent as ketone esters, they still can effectively elevate blood ketone levels into therapeutic ranges, and are significantly less expensive. They also taste better. Early versions were reported to commonly have a pronounced gastrointestinal emptying effect (a polite way of saying explosive diarrhea) but subsequent formulations seem to have diminished this side effect.

As ketone technology has evolved, there are different types of ketone salts, namely racemic and non-racemic ketone salts. There are also products that combine the ketone salts with MCT powder to enhance the elevation of BHB in the body (although again, some people's digestive systems are sensitive to concentrated MCTs). Some formulations combine the BHB with certain amino acids, which appears to provide a longer lasting elevated ketone level in the body.

One of the latest discussions about ketone salts revolves around the molecular configuration and how much of the supplemental BHB is bio-identical to what the body actually makes. There are two forms of BHB, the D and L forms. From a chemistry standpoint, that means that the spatial configuration is either a D (right hand) or an L (left hand) – think in terms of these being mirror images of each other like your hands – and the body makes the D (right hand) form. Most ketone salt products (*i.e.,* racemic ketone salts) contain both D and L forms, so there has been some concern and speculation that the body won't optimally use the BHB available, or that it's in some way not good for you. There are other experts and researchers who argue that it doesn't matter, and that the body will eventually use it or excrete it. But what this means is, some companies are focusing on creating ketones that are primarily in the D form and thus more effectively utilized by the body. These ketones are considered more "bio-identical" and therefore are more likely to be effectively used.

As always, with emerging technologies like ketone supplements, the products and formulas will evolve as the companies that create them look to compete and bring the best products to consumers. The important thing to remember is, ketone supplements can be a very quick and easy way to effectively elevate your blood ketone levels!

MCTs (Medium Chain Triglycerides)

There is another ketone supplement to discuss, and it's not especially fancy or sexy as some of the super-secret formulas in the ketone monoesters and ketone salts. It's MCT oils (such as coconut oil or commercially packaged oils) and MCT powders. MCTs are fat molecules consisting of a glycerol bound to medium chain fatty acids (meaning they have a "medium" length chain, between 6 and 12 carbon atoms in length – this is important to know, so you can assess the type of MCT you are taking, as noted below).

The reason MCTs are a popular ketogenic supplement is that certain MCTs convert very quickly and easily into ketones in your body after you consume them. In addition, they are considerably cheaper than some ketone salts and the ketone esters. Multiple studies have shown the benefits of MCT oils, and of course in most ketogenic diets, coconut oil figures prominently in the diet.

The MCTs are caproic acid (which is known as MCT C6, meaning 6 carbons in the chain), caprylic acid (C8, with 8 carbons in the chain), capric acid (C10), and lauric acid (C12). Of these, caprylic acid (C8) and capric acid (C10) convert to ketones the easiest, although many MCT products contain a fair amount of lauric acid (C12). Most aficionados of MCTs recommend looking for products with mostly caprylic acid (C8) or a combo with the majority of the product consisting of caprylic acid (C8) and capric acid (C10).

Ketone Supplements Figure Prominently in Research and Clinical Trials

The exciting thing about making a product that quickly, easily, and consistently elevates your blood ketone levels, is that a lot of research has begun testing the benefits of exogenous ketone supplements on various conditions in humans (many older studies on ketogenic compounds were done on lab rats and mice). For example, if you go to the government's Clinical Trials Registry database (www.clinicaltrials.gov) and search for "ketone supplement," "ketone monoester," or "racemic ketone salts" you will get a huge number of studies that come up that are using these compounds in their trials. This is very promising, and hopefully when the trials are completed, there will be increasingly positive evidence showing the benefits of ketone supplementation for health and disease management and therapeutics.

Some impressive research is just now beginning to hit. For example, a study released in early 2020 showed that ketone monoester supplementation help stabilize brain networks (verified by MRI and PET imaging) even when the subjects ate carbs along with the ketone supplement! The brain appears to preferentially use ketones even when glucose is present. This is groundbreaking because it means you can get the benefits of ketones by supplementation, if you can't stomach a ketogenic diet!

Over the past several years, multiple companies have come out with exogenous ketone supplements. We both personally have used and can recommend exogenous ketones. We have used MCT oil products, ketone monoesters and racemic ketone salts, which put us in a measurable state of ketosis in less than an hour. Our own experiences have been absolutely fascinating, and we can confidently recommend that people try some form of ketone supplementation to enhance their efforts to achieve and maintain ketosis. BHB is such a fascinating and valuable molecule that has so many benefits as a fuel source, signaling molecule, and biological compound that we believe ketone supplementation will soon be as commonplace as taking vitamin C or a multi-vitamin mineral supplement.

The fact is, following a ketogenic diet can be extremely challenging. As we said before, most people don't want or don't have the discipline to eat 65-75% fats and keep their carbs under 10% of their intake in order to achieve nutritional ketosis. And one misstep can throw you out of ketosis for days or even weeks. That's where the supplement comes in. You can get your body into a state of ketosis within an hour and *stay* in a heightened state of ketosis for hours by using a supplement.

Some keto purists will say it's using a short cut to do something you could or should do with diet alone. But we prefer to be realistic. People eat things intentionally or by mistake that aren't keto-friendly. They may want a cheat meal or to celebrate a birthday or big event by indulging in something sweet. With a ketone supplement, if someone goes off the diet or eats something carb-laden, they can still get the benefits of ketones without having to be in a state of strict nutritional ketosis. In addition, the diet is not for everyone, and can be difficult to follow, for example, for someone with cognitive decline, but they might benefit from using a ketone supplement. In fact, we think of ketone supplements as being "boosters" when coupled with the other techniques we discuss in this book.

In addition, many people report appetite suppression (which has been verified by research) when taking a BHB or MCT supplement, and this helps them to avoid snacking and overeating, which is key if fat loss is a goal.

The bottom line is, consuming ketones can give you many of the same benefits as the diet, and can boost the effects of ketogenic or low-carb eating. Ketones are a phenomenal health and performance supplement just by themselves. They are of course even better when combined with low carb or keto dieting, intermittent fasting, and the exercise techniques we describe in this book! Consider them as a potential part of your fitness and health toolbox.

Our goal is not to use this book to sell or promote products, but to point out what we believe are valuable supplements that can help you achieve your health and fitness goals. So we suggest you give it a try and see for yourself. Because the truth is, you don't HAVE to take a supplement to experience ketosis – you can follow the ketogenic diet, fast, and exercise – but taking a supplement can enhance your ability to get into therapeutic ketosis, and you can maintain steady ketone levels even if you aren't being as strict as you need to be to achieve pure nutritional ketosis.

In addition, supplementing with ketones while transitioning into a low-carb or ketogenic nutrition plan can help provide a high-energy fuel source and stave off keto flu and energy deficits while your body adapts to this new way of fueling itself!

What might you expect to experience? Let's check out a few benefits quickly since we discuss them at length elsewhere in the book:

Benefits of Ketosis on the Brain

The ketogenic diet has been used since the early 1900s to help control epileptic seizures in epilepsy patients and recent studies have shown it improves memory and cognitive function in dementia and Alzheimer's patients. It has also been shown to have a neuroprotective effect in cases of traumatic brain injury and anecdotally in PTSD, and has been shown to improve symptoms and enhance skills and cognition in autistic patients. Studies are being done that suggest these benefits can be extended to ALS, Parkinson's and other cognitive disorders like ADD and ADHD, and even shows potential in depression, bipolar disorders and schizophrenia.

As mentioned before, a landmark 2020 study showed that ketones could help improve cognition and stabilize brain network function caused by aging or diseases such as Alzheimer's and dementia. They may even be preventative!

Benefits of Ketosis on the Body

The list of ketones' physical benefits is impressive. The ketogenic diet causes weight and fat loss, and more importantly, it has been shown to improve diabetic symptoms, and helps improve insulin sensitivity and efficacy in the body. The ketone metabolite beta-hydroxybutyrate has also been shown to inhibit NLRP3 inflammasome activity and thus imparts an anti-inflammatory effect (anecdotal reports show individuals have received relief from rheumatoid arthritis, polycystic ovary disease, migraine headaches, eczema, and other conditions caused by inflammatory processes). They also act as signaling molecules for gene expression and help protect the body from reactive oxygen species. Finally for those seeking weight loss, ketone supplementation can help you avoid snacking and overeating because of the often-reported appetite suppressing effect of BHB.

Ketones as an Energy Source

Most people who achieve ketosis report feeling super-human like energy levels and a high level of mental cognition and focus. This may be due to the fact that ketones provide 38% more adenosine triphosphate (ATP – your mitochondria's energy source) than glucose. So the energy benefit when using ketones for fuel is significant, and when your brain uses ketones, it is essentially running on a very high-yield fuel source.

Ketones and Athletic Performance

Several studies on endurance athletes have shown that they are able to perform at a higher level for a longer period of time when in ketosis. Many recent Tour de France riders supplemented with a new ketone-based product and experienced great results. In a study of elite rowers, they achieved better overall speed and performance of a few % better than previous times, and many set personal bests. In athletes, any uptick in performance can be the difference between winning or losing, or placing or not placing.

Summary

As you can see, there are a number of ways exogenous ketones are beneficial in the body. It's up to you to decide if you want to combine supplementation with the other techniques we describe in the book to achieve and maintain ketosis. Our own personal experience is that we follow tight nutritional parameters, and use the supplemental ketones as a booster to ensure that our ketone levels are consistently in the range of therapeutic ketosis.

Getting Into Ketosis and Staying There

Method 4: Exercise

We'll cover exercise in more depth later in the book. The point we want to make in this section is that exercise is a great adjunct to help your body get into ketosis quickly and stay there. Think about it: exercise burns glucose and glycogen stores in your muscles. Once your body has exhausted those stores, it has to turn to another energy source for fuel, and we want that fuel to be fat and ketones. Now, people who follow a normal diet are eating so many carbs that they quickly and constantly replenish the glucose and glycogen that their body burns during exercise. In fact, most people probably don't exercise enough to completely use their body's stores, unless they're doing very lengthy workouts, or endurance events like triathlons or marathons. However, as soon as carbs are consumed, the body will use them to replenish those glycogen stores. For those who are not running marathons, if they are eating a standard American diet, they are overeating carbs and sugar, which are never completely burned off for energy, and that surplus energy ends up stored as fat.

Thus, if you're on a low carb, ketogenic diet, your body isn't getting lots of carbs to replenish glucose and glycogen. It HAS to turn to fat, fatty acids, and ketones for energy. If you add regular exercise and activity to the mix, you're accelerating and coaxing along the process by which your body recognizes that it doesn't have glucose or glycogen to use as fuel, and it needs to generate ketones from your dietary fat consumption, or from your body's fat stores!

Another factor is the intensity level of the exercise you are doing. If you are doing a high level of intensity when you exercise, you will burn those glycogen stores faster, which means you'll achieve ketosis faster. That high-intensity exercise really sends signals to your body that it needs fuel to accommodate this demand in energy, and if there's not enough glucose and glycogen, it'll start to look for fatty acids to convert into ketones.

Now technically, you *can* exercise your way into a low state of ketosis, but only temporarily. You'd need to do a lot of endurance work, all the time, and completely and repeatedly exhaust your glucose stores to make your body turn to your fat stores for ketogenesis. But it would be a fleeting achievement if you consumed any carbs. So we think of exercise as an adjunct – albeit a very helpful and healthy one – to encourage your body to achieve and maintain ketosis.

Therefore, we include exercise as one of our 4 methods, because when you thoughtfully and deliberately combine exercise with low-carb ketogenic dieting, intermittent fasting, and/or ketone supplementation, it will help you achieve and stay in a deep, therapeutic state of ketosis with little complexity. And, as we all know, exercise is good for you, period.

Check out the chapter on Types of Exercise later in the book for more ideas and details about what different types of exercise you might want to do, and what's most effective for fat loss, if you need some suggestions! We will also talk a little about the transition from being a glucose-burner to a fat and ketone burner, and how that my impact your exercise capacity temporarily.

Chapter 3: Common Myths and Misperceptions

As with any diet or lifestyle choice, the ketogenic method does have its detractors. Some physicians, nurses, dieticians and nutritionists, and even some celebrity fitness gurus claim that a ketogenic diet is extreme, unhealthy, or even dangerous. However, that is categorically false. The ketogenic diet is safe, effective, and is even being used by one start-up to reverse type 2 diabetes. Likewise, being in ketosis is a natural, healthy, and some would even say superior, metabolic state. In fact, we are born in a state of ketosis.

So why are "experts" so negative about keto? Often times it is because they don't actually understand it, or confuse it with other diets, or confuse ketosis with ketoacidosis (which we address below in this chapter). The sad truth is, health-care practitioners are taught very little about diets and nutrition. In fact, the physicians we speak with say they got about 1 day's worth of nutrition education in 4 years of medical school. So nutrition is not a key part of their education. Yet, we know that nutrition has a profound impact on health. So let's dig in.

Our goal in this chapter is to tackle the criticisms, misinformation, and outright lies that you might have heard about the ketogenic diet and ketogenic therapies.

MYTH #1: Ketosis is dangerous! (Ketosis vs Diabetic Ketoacidosis)

This is one of our favorites because it's a great opportunity to educate people. Ketosis and ketogenesis are natural, healthy states for the body, and ketone bodies themselves have numerous health benefits when they are produced or supplemented in normal therapeutic levels. But most healthcare professionals, nutritionists and dieticians only hear about ketones when they are taught about a dangerous and life-threatening condition called diabetic ketoacidosis (DKA), when ketone levels (and glucose levels) reach an extremely high, toxic level in the body. Ketoacidosis can occur in a diabetic patient with very high, uncontrolled blood glucose who doesn't produce insulin or is extremely insulin resistant (type 1 diabetics are more at risk of this condition; it is not as common in type 2 diabetics).

What happens is the body senses high blood glucose, which is toxic, but there is no insulin available to shuttle the glucose into the body's cells, or the patient is so insulin resistant that the insulin doesn't do its job. Even though the bloodstream is teeming with glucose, it's not getting to the cells to be used as fuel, so the body gets confused, thinking it needs fuel, and starts creating ketone bodies to be used as fuel. With all the glucose and ketones circulating in the body, it creates a vicious circle of high glucose levels and ketone body production, and the blood eventually becomes toxic and acidic. Hence the name, keto-acidosis.

Here's the thing – to get to this level of toxicity and acidity, your body has to have a very, VERY high level of ketones and glucose. A ketogenic diet, as well as ketogenic supplements, will not put a toxic level of ketones into your body, nor will it cause high levels of glucose in your body, so concerns about that happening are not warranted.

That said, if you are a type 1 diabetic with uncontrolled blood glucose, you need to monitor your glucose and ketone levels carefully, and should always talk to your medical professional about the impact of a ketogenic diet. The good news is, more and more studies are showing that a low carb or ketogenic diet, when properly administered and followed, can help type 1 diabetics too!

The other thing we think is worth pointing out is that babies are born in a state of ketosis and continue while breastfeeding (mother's milk is nature's perfect ketogenic food). In fact, it's estimated that babies and mothers are ketotic in the third trimester and at birth, and that babies' brains derive up to 30% or more of their energy from ketone bodies. So any concerns about a ketogenic diet not being safe, or ketones being toxic, should look to Mother Nature and the fact that ketosis is a normal and healthy prenatal and neonatal state.

MYTH #2: You have to eat a lot of meat/protein during a ketogenic diet

This is one of the most common misperceptions we run into when talking to people about the ketogenic diet. You don't have to eat any meat on this diet, nor do you have you eat much protein. *In fact, keto is actually a fairly low to moderate protein diet.* A well-formulated ketogenic diet should consist of 70-75% fat, 20-25% protein, and 10% or less carbohydrates (ideally 5% or less but some argue that 10% is acceptable). Therefore, keto is not risky to your kidneys nor is it a heavy protein or meat based diet. In fact, eating too much protein can knock your body out of ketosis because your body can actually convert excess protein into glucose using a process called gluconeogenesis. It's very easy to eat too much protein, which is why we recommend tracking your macros with an app like MyFitnessPal or some comparable macro tracker.

This also means that vegetarians or vegans or people who don't eat a lot of animal based products can still follow a low carb keto lifestyle – it's not necessary to eat meat to achieve ketosis.

MYTH #3: The ketogenic diet is a starvation diet

This is something we hear a lot from nutritionists and dieticians. The reality is that you do not starve yourself on a ketogenic diet. You get to eat a lot of rich, satiating foods that help you feel full, and often times you don't get hungry as often or as quickly. That's a good thing! You still eat a normal amount of calories – but they come from fats, which are more calorie dense than carbohydrates and protein. Carbs and protein have 4 calories per gram, whereas fats have 9 calories per gram. So you probably will be eating smaller portions, but that's because you're eating much more calorie-dense food.

Part of the other reason for this misconception about starvation is the way the ketogenic diet was defined in the past. To prepare for writing this book, we looked into the published research on the ketogenic diet, and noticed that in a lot of older dietary studies, when researchers used a "ketogenic diet" they did not use a diet high in fat and low in carbs. Instead, they simply used a diet extremely low in calories – a starvation diet. And the fact is, if you starve yourself, you will eventually go into ketosis. In fact many of the early studies we read used the term "starvation ketosis" **Therefore, a lot of doctors, dieticians, and nutritionists mistakenly think that the ketogenic diet equals starvation.** This is NOT true, and we now know that a well-formulated ketogenic diet still has a normal number of calories, but almost no carbs. In fact, when you look at a ketogenic diet, in a way it's tricking your body into thinking it's starving, by eliminating the glucose component – so it has no choice to switch to fat and ketones for fuel. So it's true we are technically starving the body of carbohydrates – but NOT starving in the traditional sense of the term. Avocadoes, bacon, eggs, fatty meats and fish, cheese, nuts, coconut oil, butter (real butter, not margarine) are all on the menu with a ketogenic diet!

MYTH #4: The ketogenic diet is not sustainable long-term (or it is dangerous long-term)

This is a head-scratcher. We are not sure how things like this get into people's heads. The fact is, we have a great deal of documented clinical research and science supporting the successful long-term use of the ketogenic diet. As mentioned before, the diet was used for childhood epilepsy as far back as the 1920s and many patients were on the diet for years (even decades), without significant side effects – other than relieving their epilepsy, which was the desired side effect!! We postulate that the idea that it's not safe or healthy long-term probably stemmed from the previous disproven fact that people either associated it with starvation (as discussed in Myth #3 above) or due to the misconception that fats are bad for you. Which leads us to the next one...

MYTH #5: Eating a lot of fat is bad for you

We probably should have put this as #1 since it's the first thing people say when you suggest they eat a diet that's 70% fat! The fact is, fats are extremely healthy for you (we mean saturated fats, not trans-fats). Your body needs saturated fat and cholesterol to operate optimally and efficiently. Your brain is 60% fat and cholesterol!! Your body also requires fat to create hormones, and

Chapter 3: Common Myths and Misperceptions

for a properly functioning nervous system. Cholesterol, also vilified, is a substance your body uses to repair inflamed and damaged tissues. So avoiding fat and cholesterol is in reality not healthy, which is exactly the opposite of what "the experts" have been telling us since the 1950s and 60s.

How did this happen? Well it was a combination of bad science, politics, and influence by the sugar and food industry. It turns out that the early research by scientist Ancel Keys that pointed the finger at saturated fat as the cause of heart disease was dead wrong. Over the past several decades, as the Western world moved to a supposedly "healthy" diet low in saturated fat and high in carbohydrates, the rates of obesity, diabetes and heart disease have skyrocketed. Not long ago, it was discovered that Keys ignored and omitted entire populations of data that would have disproven his hypothesis that saturated fat caused heart disease. Sadly, instead of debunking his claim, his inaccurate published work became the basis for the modern nutritional guidelines that have caused much of the population's health to plummet.

It turns out that the key issue in heart disease is inflammation (which is discussed at much greater length elsewhere in this book, as well as in Dr. Lori's book *How To Fight FATflammation"*). You see, fat and cholesterol don't clog your arteries the way bacon grease can clog your kitchen sink pipes. The human body is much more complex than that. What actually happens is that when your blood vessels become damaged due to inflammation and other causes, the body dispatches cholesterol molecules as part of the healing process. Under normal healthy conditions, that cholesterol would do its part to help repair your damaged blood vessels. But when inflammation, free radicals, and reactive oxygen species are present, cholesterol molecules can become oxidized and can penetrate and adhere to the blood vessel walls and begin forming arterial plaques. That's the bad part – and it's the inflammation that's responsible, not the cholesterol. Don't blame cholesterol for what the sugar and bread did! And yet we have, unfortunately.

Of course, one of the primary causes of systemic inflammation in the body is consumption of sugar and simple or processed carbohydrates, which convert to blood glucose (sugar), which results in your body releasing large quantities of insulin. Both glucose and insulin are inflammatory. So the ketogenic diet can be beneficial because it greatly reduces your consumption of sugar and carbs that would become blood glucose, and therefore, your body does not experience the levels of insulin release that it would if you were fueling yourself on sugar and carbs.

In addition, recent research has shown that ketone bodies (specifically beta-hydroxybutyrate, or BHB) have been shown to have an anti-inflammatory effect by inhibiting certain inflammasomes (inflammatory signaling platforms in the body, which start the entire inflammatory process), so the good news is that ketosis can be protective to your body, in addition to the many other benefits it provides. Thus, we can completely de-bunk the myths that the ketogenic diet and eating fat are bad for you – they are in fact quite healthy for you.

Myth #6: Your body and brain require carbohydrates so keto has to be bad for you

This is another example of misinformation being used to smear a very healthy way of eating. The fact is, your body can run and function perfectly without you eating a single gram of carbs. While it's true the there are some bodily functions that require glucose, your body can create its own glucose molecules from proteins by a process called gluconeogenesis. So there is no physical or physiologic requirement to consume carbohydrates. In fact, new research is showing that too much glucose may actually be detrimental to brain network function and activity as we age, whereas ketones repair brain network function.

Summary

The bottom line is that there are a lot of critics and detractors of ketosis and the ketogenic diet, but most of the negativity is simply due to misunderstandings or a lack of the facts. We hope this chapter helps to clarify some of the common objections and concerns people have – and puts your mind at ease about them. Even though keto is gaining mainstream popularity and is being talked about everywhere, we still see and read "experts" who parrot the old outdated dogma that eating fats are bad, and that keto is simply an unhealthy fad for speedy weight loss. As you are learning through this book, keto is the key to unlocking a whole level of health that you may have never thought was possible!

THE KETOGENIC KEY

SECTION II:

THE BENEFITS OF KETOSIS ON METABOLIC DISEASES

Section II: The Benefits of Ketosis on Metabolic Diseases

Chapter 4. Keto and Weight Loss and Fat Loss (Obesity)

What do celebrities like Gwyneth Paltrow, LeBron James, Kim Kardashian, and Halle Berry have in common? They have all at one time touted and attributed their lean physiques to the ketogenic diet – and for good reason. The ketogenic diet transforms overweight individuals using a nutritional plan that features mostly fat, moderate protein and very low carbohydrate intake.

The average person has about 40,000 calories worth of fat stored throughout our bodies, and some people have even more. Back in our caveman days when carbohydrates were not readily available (except for seasonally available berries or honey), our ancestors were forced to use their fat stores for energy as a result of food scarcity. This fat was mobilized by their bodies and converted into ketones, which are the body's natural alternative fuel source. Ketones are also a much cleaner-burning source of fuel that just happen to provide a plethora of beneficial health effects, including fat and weight loss. You see, the ketogenic diet coaxes our body to use fat as fuel, rather than storing it on our bodies. And when done properly, it will use the fat already stored on our bodies for fuel, making us thinner, leaner, and healthier. Weight loss (and more specifically, fat loss) is often a side effect of ketosis.

In one study, people on a ketogenic diet lost 2.2 times more weight than those on a low-calorie, low-fat diet. Triglyceride and HDL cholesterol levels also improved among the ketogenic dieters. This is indicative of a diet that one does not feel deprived on, where it's not controlled or restrictive, but allows one to consume plenty of delicious and healthy foods that feed one's metabolism.

The Metabolic Disease Epidemic

Sadly, obesity and metabolic diseases (diabetes, heart disease and related disorders) have become the world's biggest health problems. In fact, at least 2.8 million adults die from obesity-related causes each year – which means that 7,671 people die **each day** from these easily preventable and treatable conditions! To combat these diseases, many people are using the ketogenic diet, which has been shown to powerfully transform one's weight and health. Even better news is that the ketogenic diet is backed by robust research, unlike typical "fad diets" out there, of which few are actually supported by science.

Metabolic Syndrome is also rampant now affecting over 50 million people and this is no surprise as it is closely linked to obesity and even just being overweight. What is Metabolic Syndrome? It's a cluster of conditions such as increased blood pressure, high blood sugar, excess body fat around the waist and organs, and abnormal cholesterol or triglyceride levels— these conditions typically occur together, increasing your risk of – and often resulting in – heart disease, stroke and diabetes.

Fighting Metabolic Disease With Ketosis

The main goal of the ketogenic diet is to put your body into a state of ketosis, which means your body is taking fat and turning it into ketones to circulate throughout your body as a cellular super fuel. This is a very natural metabolic reaction that happens when we burn fat for fuel, instead of carbs and glucose. The more fat you eat, the less cravings, hunger and desire to nibble you will have. On the ketogenic diet, you'll find that eating fatty foods will keep you satiated and not prone to snacking.

By eating a larger amount of fat, and very little carbohydrates, we are basically eliminating or greatly reducing the amount of glucose (sugar) being consumed. Without access to glucose, a quick and easy-to-burn fuel, the body has no other choice than to utilize your fat stores for energy. It does this through the liver, which converts fatty acids from your diet or body fat stores into ketones for the body and brain to use as fuel. This keeps blood sugar levels stable and your insulin low. Your body then sheds the excess weight as it uses fats to maintain itself.

Therefore, the key to the ketogenic diet is eating plenty of fat. Many people often confuse the ketogenic diet with the "Atkins Diet" which was very popular in the 1970s. Atkins was a little similar to keto, and it did promote achieving ketosis to drive weight loss. One major distinction between the two, however, is that the Atkins Diet promoted consuming a lot of protein, whereas the ketogenic diet recommends moderate to low protein consumption. Large amounts of protein are believed to tax the liver causing inflammation, and stress the kidneys. Therefore, consuming high fat, not high protein, is a Ketogenic Key.

Here are general mechanisms that help to promote weight loss on the ketogenic diet:

- Reduction in carbohydrates
- Increase in healthy fats
- Moderate protein intake
- Appetite suppressant - a direct hunger-reducing role of ketone bodies—the body's main fuel source on the diet.
- Improved insulin sensitivity
- Decreased fat storage due to reduced lipogenesis
- Increased fat-burning
- Decrease in appetite-stimulating hormones, such as insulin and ghrelin, and increased sensitivity to satiety hormones such as leptin

Smoothing Out The Weight Loss Roller Coaster

Have you had the roller coaster experience of weight loss? You temporarily lose weight, then gain it back, and you're back to the drawing board. The challenge of losing weight and keeping it off can be discouraging and frustrating for many. The good news is that research shows with the ketogenic diet, the weight comes off and stays off.

<u>Muscle Mass</u>

Chapter 4. Keto and Weight Loss and Fat Loss (Obesity)

Part of the reason for this is that the ketogenic diet helps your body maintain muscle mass. One of the side effects of low-calorie diets is the loss of lean muscle mass, which is a problem for long-term and sustained weight loss, because muscle mass is important for maintaining a sound metabolism – the more muscle mass you have, the higher your metabolism will run.

Appetite

Our bodies have built-in sensors that keep us "energy balanced" for our own protection; should food become scarce, our metabolic signals kick in. However, with obesity and metabolic diseases such as type 2 diabetes, these signals are altered and sometimes muted, making weight loss even more difficult.

Appetite is one of those key signals that factors into weight gain and weight loss. When our appetite is sated, we eat less, and the weight comes off more easily because we are not consuming as many calories. What's very interesting is that the appetite buffering effects are a result of the anti-inflammatory properties of nutritional ketosis. This research goes hand-in-hand with what Dr. Lori discusses in her book *How To Fight FATflammation.* Research shows that it is ketosis that promotes weight loss by mitigating appetite combined with easier access to using stored fat for fuel.

Hormones

Hormones are also integral signalers and factors of why fat loss is successfully achieved with the ketogenic diet. We have hormones at play that essentially direct our fat loss. In addition to the fat storage hormone insulin, and the hunger hormone ghrelin, there is the satiety hormone leptin. Leptin is secreted by the fat cells, and it tells the brain when you've had enough to eat.

The issue with these hormones is that your body can become **resistant** to them. You see, when we consume a lot of carbohydrates repeatedly during the day, we have constant blood sugar spikes, which result in repeatedly high levels of circulating insulin. Remember, insulin signals the body to engage in fat storage. So when you become resistant to insulin, its levels build up, further prompting your body into storing fat. That can dovetail into leptin resistance, which means your brain is not getting the signal you've had enough to eat. Being resistant to leptin is another key driver of obesity and weight gain. The more body fat one carries, the more leptin is produced. Eventually the body becomes resistant to "listening" to the leptin signals, and thus the hungrier we become! So as you can see, hormones that control appetite (ghrelin), fat storage (insulin) and hunger (leptin) get completely out of kilter when we eat lots and lots of carbohydrates and sugar.

Ketosis to the rescue! Leptin resistance, insulin resistance, increased appetite and resulting weight gain will become a thing of the past when we achieve ketosis. Nutritional ketosis can balance out these hormones, and eliminate resistance, which enhances appetite control, reduces inflammation and makes it easy to maintain a healthy weight, while enjoying delicious and satiating foods.

Section II: The Benefits of Ketosis on Metabolic Diseases

Chapter 5. Keto and Managing and Reversing Type 2 Diabetes

"So long as we have other sources of energy, humans do not need carbohydrates. The minimum daily carbohydrate requirement to sustain life is zero! We may enjoy them, but they are not necessary for life."

~Dr. Stephen Phinney, Virta Health

The Diabetes Epidemic

Chances are you already know that type 2 diabetes is a global epidemic, and its statistics are rising rapidly. In fact, diabetes rates have quadrupled since 1980. More than *100 million* U.S. adults are now living with diabetes or pre-diabetes. What is worse is that 84 million, or 1 out of 3 Americans, have pre-diabetes and 90% of those people do not realize they have this condition.

If there is no intervention, diabetes will affect over half the population by 2025, a staggering statistic because this disease is a horrible one for patients and their families and an expensive one for all of us as well as our healthcare system.

Diabetes is a disease of glucose intolerance and insulin deficiency or resistance. You see, glucose is a fuel that feeds your body's cells, but to enter your cells it needs the hormone insulin. Insulin is a key player in the two different types of diabetes: type 1 and type 2. People with type 1 diabetes do not produce insulin. People with type 2 diabetes don't respond to insulin optimally and later in the disease process, often don't make enough insulin. The problem with not making insulin, or having your body fail to respond to insulin, is that it creates high blood glucose levels, which are both toxic and inflammatory. To complicate this, insulin is also inflammatory. So diabetes is a disease wherein the problem (too much glucose in the bloodstream) causes an inflammatory state, and the current medical intervention (injecting insulin) reduces the blood glucose levels, but also contributes to the inflammatory environment in a patient's body.

Before we delve into this, let's take a look at how we got ourselves into this epidemic of obesity and diabetes.

What Went Wrong?

For almost 40 years (since 1980), the U.S. government has recommended that Americans increase carbohydrate intake and absolutely avoid fats. Despite this advice, Americans have become fatter and sicker than ever before. The following graphic shows the rise in obesity in the US, as well as how it correlates to the US government's dietary guidelines released in 1980. The spike is undeniable:

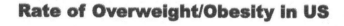

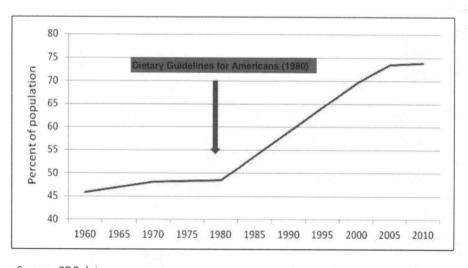

Source: CDC data

Chapter 5. Keto and Managing and Reversing Type 2 Diabetes

However, the good news is that there's hope. What many individuals do not know is that pre-diabetes and type 2 diabetes can be prevented and *reversed,* or put into a state of remission naturally.

Many believe that diabetes is genetic, or runs in families, and that if your mother or father had diabetes, you are destined to have it as well.   That idea is completely false. Even with all of the new scientific research refuting this concept, diabetes being hereditary is still an old, outdated and entrenched idea with some doctors and other health professionals.

The old diabetes dogma, an often misunderstood and/or the rooted older mindset, is that type 2 diabetes is predominantly an inherited disease or a self-afflicted one that cannot be reversed, and can only be *managed.* The current best practice in diabetes management is to use drugs that only maintain or in some cases even worsen the disease.   The drugs simply do not work to address the core problem, and the diabetes is then labeled "chronic and progressive." Over time, as patients rely on and continually use these inflammatory medications, the disease does in fact often get worse, not better.

The existing treatments are essentially based on misguided information, and characterize one of the biggest criticisms of our existing healthcare system, which is that it is reactionary not preventative, and typically treats the symptoms of a disease, rather than addressing the core, underlying cause(s) of a disease. **What scientists and nutrition visionaries have recently realized is that type 2 diabetes is NOT an incurable disease, and it can not only be managed, but it can actually be reversed – with nutritional and lifestyle changes.**

One great example of this is when a diabetic patient loses weight, often times their type 2 diabetes will greatly improve, and in some cases even go away. So you see, it doesn't make sense that type 2 diabetes should get worse and worse if insulin or other medications were the answer. Instead, let me repeat that it is a disease that can be mitigated and reversed with nutrition and diet as the focus, rather than drugs. And as you can guess, the ketogenic diet has been shown to do exactly that – it can greatly improve, and even reverse, diabetes.

Virta Health (www.virtahealth.com) is an excellent example of an organization that has used nutrition and lifestyle changes to successfully reverse type 2 diabetes. In their year-long clinical trial of 262 patients, they showed the adoption of a low-carb, high-fat keto diet and other lifestyle changes resulted in markedly reduced need for insulin and other medications in more than 60% of the participants. In other words, they were able to significantly reduce the amount of medication they needed. In addition, many of the patients actually saw complete reversal of their diabetes. The reason this is so groundbreaking is that it proves that lifestyle and nutrition can solve the diabetes dilemma, and it de-bunks the dogma that diabetes is a life-long disease that one must continually manage with medication. It turns out, from what the latest research is showing us, that the exact opposite is true.

The research by Virta Health also showed that the ketone body beta-hydroxybutyrate (BHB) dramatically reduced oxidative stress and inflammation, which in turn reduced the root cause of insulin resistance (diabetes). So ketones can be a key player in the treatment of diabetes. The challenge is overcoming the decades-old belief that the best way to treat diabetes is with insulin and drugs, rather than reverse the underlying cause.

> *"What scientists and nutrition visionaries have recently realized is that type 2 diabetes is NOT an incurable disease, and it can not only be managed, but it can actually be reversed – with nutritional and lifestyle changes."*

Why is treating diabetes with insulin a problem? Because type 2 diabetes is essentially a result of too much circulating blood sugar and insulin in the body, yet, the cells cannot receive any more. As Jason Fung, MD author of *The Obesity Code* states: "When you give more insulin, it is like treating an alcoholic with more alcohol. The symptoms such as tremors will go away for a period of time." The same is true for those with type 2 diabetes, when you give them insulin, their blood sugars look better, but the diabetes gradually worsens, because insulin and continually elevated blood glucose continue to create an inflammatory cellular environment, especially in the vascular system and blood vessels.

"No drug can do this. Diet is a much more potent tool"

Chapter 5. Keto and Managing and Reversing Type 2 Diabetes

~Dr. Steven Phinney

This is exactly where a ketogenic key comes in. If the problem is a vicious circle of eating carbohydrates, which causes high blood sugar and requires high levels of insulin, it follows that a low-carbohydrate diet should be a first line approach. A low-carb diet like the ketogenic diet will keep blood sugar levels low to begin with. When your blood sugar level is low, or stable, you do not need insulin to shuttle glucose into the cells, thus breaking that vicious cycle. To do this we can use multiple powerful approaches: the ketogenic diet, intermittent fasting, and ketone supplementation, individually or in combination.

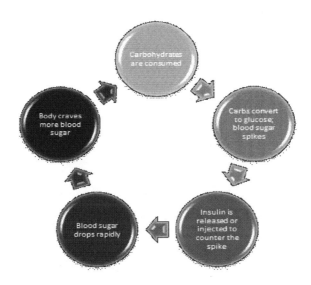

Figure: Vicious circle of carbohydrate consumption, blood glucose spikes, and insulin release, leading to cravings for more carbohydrate consumption.

The ketogenic diet will reduce the amount of carbohydrate (sugar) intake and prevent chronically high blood glucose and reduce or eliminate the big insulin spikes. In a diabetic's case, this translates to the need for injecting large quantities of insulin or taking insulin-mimicking drugs.

Intermittent fasting, spacing the time between your meals (discussed in detail elsewhere in this book), will also lower blood sugar and keep the levels stable.

Ketone supplementation has also been recently shown in a clinical trial to decrease and stabilize blood glucose levels, event when a person is consuming carbohydrates in their diet.

What about exercise? Well, it turns out that diet is the primary tool to fight T2D, and exercise is a secondary player – and useful. Exercise can help burn off excess glucose and help cells become much more insulin sensitive. So there is definitely a role for exercise. Exercise alone will not necessarily lead to diabetes management or reversal if a person is still consuming a lot of carbs and has chronically high blood glucose. But a ketogenic, low-carb diet in combination with exercise can be a powerful and effective one-two punch!

The bottom line is that diabetes is not a life-sentence. It can be managed, halted, improved, and even reversed. It all starts with what a type 2 diabetic eats. A large multi-country panel of endocrinology and nutrition experts put out a guideline in 2015 that called for dietary carbohydrate restriction to be the first line therapy for type 2 diabetes. Sadly, it hardly seems to have gained much traction in most healthcare-oriented dietary recommendations. But that is changing, and we will continue to spread this low-carb gospel to help diabetics who are struggling to manage their disease, its symptoms and its repercussions on their health.

Section II: The Benefits of Ketosis on Metabolic Diseases

Chapter 6. Keto and Heart Disease

"What right has the federal government to propose that the American people conduct a vast nutritional experiment, with themselves as subjects, on the strength of so little evidence?"

~Dr. Phillip Handler, the former president of the U.S. National Academy of Sciences

It is a tragedy and grim statistic: more than 610,000 Americans will die from heart disease this year. Every 40 seconds, someone in the United States has a heart attack. It's the leading cause of death for both men and women. Why? For decades, doctors, health professionals, nutritionists and others have prescribed a diet low in fat, and particularly low in saturated fat. It was thought that foods high in this type of fat would clog arteries and cause heart disease. Yet, even though nutritional guidelines have recommended against eating saturated fats, and United States citizens have followed this advice, they have continued to get fatter, sicker, and have increased incidence and death caused by heart disease. As the quote by Dr. Handler above points out, this has been a failed nutritional experiment, and the American people have suffered the consequences with their health, and for too many, their lives.

How Did This Tragedy Happen?

Presently, and it has been a slow transformation, the tide is turning away from the current popular ideas against saturated fat and cholesterol consumption. But how did we get there?

It all began with Ancel Keys, an American scientist, and his **Seven Countries Study** published in 1953, which concluded that consumption of saturated fat caused heart disease. Although it was not immediately realized at the time, there were two main flaws with this study: (1) correlation does not equal causation; and (2) cherry-picking of the data.

What do we mean by "correlation does not equal causation?"

This is a common mistake made in comparing data from different groups and associating a specific common thing with a certain outcome. It may have a correlation, but it doesn't mean that it *caused* the outcome. Just because two things happen in the same group of people, doesn't mean one caused the other.

For example, let's say in a group of 1,000 people, 2% of them ate eggs almost every day. And in that 2%, a large group of them also had cancer. It would be a huge leap of logic to assume that eating eggs caused the cancer. Were other risk factors taking into account? Did they smoke? Did they consume lots of processed foods, or have diabetes or work in jobs where they were exposed to carcinogens? Yet this is the type of "causation" that researchers report on all the time. What if the majority of that 2% wore white socks. Wouldn't it be ridiculous to then say that wearing white socks causes cancer? Of course!

So when we say correlation does not equal causation, this is the type of "jumping to conclusions" that we mean. In dietary studies especially, this type of "correlation" is reported all the time, which is why we've seen complete reversals and contradictions about whether we should eat certain types of foods, like eggs. So, it's very irresponsible to try to push the agenda that a certain correlation is in fact the cause of a certain outcome.

What do we mean by cherry-picking the data?

In the case of Ancel Keys' Seven Countries Study, data for 22 countries was readily available to him, but he only used the data from the 7 countries that confirmed his personally biased beliefs about causation. This allowed Keys to make the large leap of logic that a diet high in saturated fat is a direct cause of high cholesterol in the blood, which causes heart disease.

The American Heart Association initially did not agree with Keys, yet, without *any* controlled trial to prove Keys' hypotheses, the AHA, in 1961, recommended reducing saturated fat and cholesterol from foods that actually help to optimize health (such as butter, fatty meats, egg yolks, and full-fat milk) and replacing them with no-fat or low fat equivalents and inflammatory processed vegetable and seed oils.

They touted that the "savior" for our heart health was a diet that was low in fat and high in carbohydrates; and in fact, the government also recommended this for decades as the basis of the USDA Food Pyramid and "MyPlate" guidelines, which further entrenched these erroneous recommendations. This mistaken prescriptive advice, along with organizations such as the AHA advocating and promoting that erroneous advice, has been a crucial element to contributing to the enormous number of heart disease cases and deaths, and the epidemic of obesity, diabetes, and metabolic disease that we are now seeing.

Currently, research clearly shows the low fat, no cholesterol advice was plain wrong; **for the majority of people, it is the over-consumption of carbohydrates (especially refined sugar and processed simple carbohydrates), not fat, that is the true underlying cause of heart disease.**

Despite the latest research, the Ancel Keys legacy is lingering. Do you love eggs? Most people do, and yet they believe that eating foods high in cholesterol such as eggs, bacon, red meat, and even fat in general, is a fast track to heart disease and poor health, because that's what has been drilled into their mind for decades. You've probably heard the expression that fatty foods are a "heart attack waiting to happen." That is what many people think when they look at a plate of eggs and bacon. Sadly, this belief, which has been held so tightly for so long, is just plain wrong, and exactly the opposite of the truth: saturated fats are in fact, quite good for you.

Consider The Prospective Urban Rural Epidemiology (PURE) study published in *The Lancet* in 2017, which studied nutrition among more than 135,000 people across 18 different countries — making it the largest-ever observational study of its kind. The researchers found that those who ate the least saturated fat had the highest rates of heart disease and mortality. And people who consumed the most saturated fat had the lowest rate of strokes.

The old no fat, no saturated fat, low-fat myth unfortun
very sadly, is still pervasive. Most people, if they are eve
nutrition labels, will first zero in on the calories and fat grams – yet
neither is as important as the quality of the food (and fat) we eat.
There is a vast difference in the way the body metabolizes 100
calories of red meat vs a 100 calorie candy bar.

Show Me the Money?

In addition to the fact that some large organizations uphold the old,
entrenched beliefs and poor quality research conclusions
regarding saturated fat – such as the already mentioned American
Heart Association and the American Diabetes Association
(although recently the ADA has begun to modify its
recommendations) – there are others who have a potentially
biased hand in perpetuating these outdated beliefs, including
pharmaceutical companies that have significant amounts of money
at stake, especially with drugs like metformin and insulin for
diabetics, and cholesterol-lowering products such as statins. They
need people with concerns about "high cholesterol" in order to
support their bottom line.

Pharmaceutical companies make money by treating people with
diseases, and so there is no financial motivation for them to make
people think they can improve a disease through diet alone. Paired
with that is the fact that our healthcare system is more focused on
treatment of problems after they manifest, than it is on preventing
them in the first place. As a result, medical professionals are
educated more about using drugs to treat conditions, rather than to
look for a nutritional or dietary solution. To complicate this, many
organizations that provide education to physicians are subsidized
by educational grants from pharmaceutical companies – even
though there are rules against direct influence of content of
education, in many clinical areas, the focus of the education is
skewed toward pharmaceutical interventions. Nutrition and diet
are almost never mentioned or considered in most therapeutic
clinical guidelines. Part of this is complicated by the unreliable data
collection methods and weak evidence found in most nutritional
research, which has made making definitive recommendations
about diet very controversial, and could potentially be
embarrassing to organizations when a complete reversal is shown

later.

Even more disturbing is that recently, evidence emerged that the sugar industry had paid scientists in the 1960s to implicate saturated fat, and minimize concerns about sugar, as a cause for heart disease. The combination of sugar and carbohydrates is the "heart attack waiting to happen" and not the vilified steak, eggs or bacon – but there have been and still are strong lobbies pushing to keep the status quo, and to even obscure the real cause of these diseases.

Is it true that companies pay to have research manipulated in their favor benefitting their bottom line? Yes. A great example of this is the POM Wonderful pomegranate juice company who was caught showing that they paid 35 million dollars for studies that conveniently concluded that drinking their POM Wonderful pomegranate juice and taking their supplements could treat, prevent or reduce the risk of heart disease, cancer and more.

The food industry also has a lot of money riding on the old low-fat dietary dogma. It is stunning to think that there are still manufacturers that use the marketing term "low fat" on their products in this day and age. If you are old enough to remember the low-fat Snackwells cookies, low-fat Entenmann's bakery goods, and almost every other processed food product out there that carried a "low-fat" label on it, you will also remember how we all gobbled it up without questioning the impact upon our health. Sadly, that impact was that we got fatter and unhealthier by eating "low fat."

How a Low Carbohydrate Intake (and Ketones) Will Protect Your Heart

Contrary to what most people think, we now truly know how to prevent heart disease. **To date there is NO conclusive evidence linking saturated fat as independent risk factor with heart disease.** As mentioned previously in the book, it is not saturated fat, it is not steak, eggs, bacon or lard that causes cardiovascular disease; instead, it is a high carbohydrate intake, particularly when combined with refined carbohydrates such as sugar, that leads to heart disease.

The ketogenic diet, which is low in carbohydrates and high in fat, is an excellent way of eating to protect oneself against heart disease. The mistaken belief that fats cause heart disease stems from weak, outdated research. The reason keto works is because it keeps carbohydrate intake low, and therefore, minimizes the chances for the inflammatory process that leads to heart and vascular disease. In addition, the ketone beta-hydroxybutyrate suppresses certain types of inflammation.

The ketogenic diet, when followed long-term, can help decrease the level of triglycerides, LDL (bad) cholesterol, and blood glucose, and increase the level of HDL (good) cholesterol. HDL cholesterol is essentially like a broom that sweeps away the bad LDL cholesterol and it, in particular, has been shown to increase markedly on a ketogenic diet.

When you are in ketosis, good things happen, such as weight loss and the reduction of inflammation, which translates to a healthy heart for life. In fact, the ketogenic diet has been shown to reverse metabolic syndrome, which is a cluster of diseases such as high blood pressure, non-alcoholic fatty liver, high blood sugar, high triglycerides, and large waist circumference, all of which are factors associated with heart disease.

How does the ketogenic diet accomplish all of this?

Mostly by replacing carbs with healthy fats like coconut oil, animal fats, nuts, avocados, olive oil, and quality meats and fish.

Fatty Acids, Ketones, and Heart Function

Recently, research has turned up some additional information about heart function and heart muscle energy metabolism. It has long been known that the preferred fuel for the heart muscle is fatty acids, although the heart muscle cells can quickly adapt to burn all sort of fuel substrates when necessary. So eating fat may be important for heart health – exactly the opposite of what our "experts" have been telling us for years. In fact, some studies have shown that increasing certain types of fatty acids helps recover heart pump activity in models of cardiac ischemia and reperfusion (when heart muscle is impaired, and suffers a lack of blood and oxygen, and then when blood flow resumes, it causes tissue injury). In models of heart failure, researchers have found that the heart will switch to ketones as fuel to help it generate energy to offset the failure process. Although this area of study is somewhat new, there are hypotheses that ketones are called upon to help the heart muscle continue to work in times of heart failure.

The Benefits of Cholesterol (Yes, Cholesterol!)

Cholesterol is highly beneficial to our health, despite all the negative press it has received over the past 40 years. Yes, saturated fat filled foods such as butter, whole eggs, coconut oil and liver, which are cholesterol dense, are now known to help play a prominent role in optimizing our health.

It is gratifying to know that cholesterol is becoming less of the devil in terms of our health. National publications, such as *Time Magazine* are even giving cholesterol its day in the sun.

However, it is important to make the distinction between unprocessed cholesterol from natural sources vs. oxidized (damaged) cholesterol. It is this damaged cholesterol that promotes the buildup of plaque in the arteries leading to atherosclerosis or clogged arteries.

> *"Accusing saturated fat and cholesterol for hardening of the arteries is like accusing white blood cells of causing infection, rather than helping the immune system address it."*
> *~Dr. Meyer Texon MD, renowned pathologist*

What are the benefits of cholesterol?
- Cholesterol is necessary for optimum hormone health and balance, and is needed to make hormones such as testosterone, progesterone, DHEA and estrogen
- Cholesterol is protective and acts as an antioxidant throughout the body
- Cholesterol is crucial for proper functioning of the brain. In fact, statins (cholesterol lowering drugs) remove cholesterol from the brain, which may be problematic
- Cholesterol is necessary for serotonin (what we refer to as the

"happy transmitter") receptors, which has a marked effect on mood
- Cholesterol is critical for repairs in our body and why, as we age, cholesterol tends to rise

To determine if the ketogenic diet is improving your cholesterol levels, have your doctor check your total-to-HDL cholesterol ratio — this is one of the best predictors of cardiovascular disease risk. Make sure your total-to-HDL cholesterol ratio is between 3 and 4.

An important caveats however, would include: if you are at risk for high levels of LDL cholesterol (i.e., levels over 400), along with high triglycerides (which can be a risk factor for heart disease and serious liver issues) and high inflammation – for example, if you have an inherited condition called "familial hypercholesterolemia" that affects up to 10% of people worldwide. People with this condition tend to experience very high cholesterol, triglycerides and inflammatory markers in response to a high-fat diet including foods such as coconut oil, butter, fatty fish, fatty meats, eggs, etc. If you are not sure whether you have this health condition, you should have your doctor administer a cholesterol test before embarking on the ketogenic diet.

Remember, though, that in 90% of the population, foods have a negligible impact upon cholesterol levels and in the vast majority, eating healthy fats will actually improve blood lipid markers such as cholesterol ratios and triglyceride levels. But there is a percentile that may have a condition such as hypercholesterolemia and therefore, consulting with your physician is always a good idea. Just make sure your doctor is informed on the latest nutritional dogma and not clinging to the old mindset that fat is bad and carbs are good!

The combination of a very healthy ketogenic diet with a lot of veggies (they add critical minerals and anti-oxidants), eggs, seafood, meat, poultry, healthy fats (which improve cholesterol), avocados, coconut oil, olive oil plus intermittent fasting, can help heal the heart and vascular systems and help to eventually come off statins and other medications, with the help of your doctor.

Who knew that eating delicious, healthful and fatty foods would protect your heart for life? Well they do – and a ketogenic diet is an

Chapter 7. Keto and Lowering Blood Pressure

excellent way of eating for these kinds of health benefits.

Section II: The Benefits of Ketosis

Chapter 7. Keto and Lowering Blood Pressure

Has your doctor told you to reduce your blood pressure? If so, you're not alone. Many individuals have this chronic condition. According to the American Heart Association, nearly 80 million American adults (almost 1 in 3!) have high blood pressure. But it doesn't have to be that way.

The ketogenic diet, and just being in the state of ketosis, are both beneficial for many areas of our health, such as reversing diabetes, reducing inflammation, improving brain health, and fat loss. What many do not realize is that keto can also improve high blood pressure. Being overweight or obese is a major trigger for high blood pressure. In fact, obesity and hypertension generally go hand-in-hand. Because ketosis and the keto diet often lead to weight loss, they also help to reduce blood pressure.

Fat versus Carbs—What Really Makes You Pack on the Pounds?

The ketogenic diet, and other low carb diets, can have a direct effect on blood pressure, primarily through their powerful ability to reduce inflammation and promote weight loss. If you are interested in lowering blood pressure, a ketogenic diet with 50 or fewer grams of carbohydrates per day may be an effective method.

Inflammation is the core underlying cause of most illness, disease, weight gain and faster-aging, and so simply removing the excess glucose and insulin stemming from all those goodies, sugar and unhealthy processed foods that people are gobbling up, will in turn, reduce the low-level inflammation that can jack up your blood pressure.

Chapter 7. Keto and Lowering Blood Pressure

In addition, research from Yale have shown that the ketone body beta-hydroxybutyrate (BHB) has a marked impact on NLRP3-inflammasome mediated inflammation. So just being in ketosis, and having elevated levels of ketones in your blood, may also help to quell that low-level inflammation in your body.

In a randomized controlled trial, which is considered top tier in research quality, headed by William S. Yancy, Jr., MD MHSc, Associate Professor in the Department of Medicine at Duke University Medical Center, showed that a low-carbohydrate ketogenic diet with exercise was more effective in lowering blood pressure compared to a low-fat diet combined with the weight-loss drug Orlistat and regular exercise. This is a remarkable finding in showing that a ketogenic diet can significantly reduce your blood pressure.

Most dietary guidelines have been massively, cleverly, unfairly, or unscrupulously put forth by the very industries responsible for the obesity epidemic (and obesity or weight gain's own cluster of health conditions such as hypertension) – by the sugar and processed food industries! Eating these high-carbohydrate foods, including processed, refined foods, subjects your body, your cells, to an over-abundance heart-harming fats, waist-widening sugar, inflammatory oils, and appetite-inducing additives.

We do know that your lifestyle can affect your risk of developing it. You are at a higher risk if you are overweight, eat an inflammatory diet such as the very sad Standard American Diet (SAD) or a highly processed diet, if you are sedentary, if drink too much, and if have other factors such as aging, ethnicity and family history.

Remember that your health conditions including hypertension can potentially be healed by taking charge of your overall health, and getting into ketosis by following a ketogenic diet, doing intermittent fasting, and/or ketone supplementation is an excellent way to start.

One thing to note: if you have high blood pressure, and are on medication for it, be sure to monitor your blood pressure and talk to your doctor. The ketogenic diet can lower your blood pressure pretty rapidly (some people report significant declines within a month or two), and if you continue to take blood pressure medication while your blood pressure becomes normal due to the diet, the medication can actually cause low blood pressure. So as always, monitor your vitals and talk to your doctor about your dietary changes.

SECTION III: BENEFITS OF KETOSIS ON INFLAMMATION AND INFLAMMATORY DISEASES

Chapter 8. Ketosis is Anti-Inflammatory

Question: **What causes inflammation?**
Answer: **Poor food choices and lifestyle factors**

If you knew you could make some changes in your life and prevent a myriad of health conditions, including diabetes, heart disease, stroke, Alzheimer's disease or arthritis, would you make those changes? What we've learned about health, inflammation and longevity in this last decade is nothing short of astonishing. Inflammation is at the core-center of many of these diseases' causes and prevention (we'll explain this paradox shortly). And, not surprisingly, some of the most impactful preventative measures we can take are nutrition related – and one showing the most promise is achieving a state of ketosis, most often via the ketogenic diet.

There is a link between inflammation and/or health conditions and weight gain that affect most people, but can also be prevented, mitigated and even reversed by addressing this incendiary player through diet and other lifestyle factors.

One of the beneficial aspects of being in ketosis is how it can be anti-inflammatory, and many people are turning to ketosis as a way to help manage and reduce symptoms from inflammation.

Let's start off by saying that we all have inflammation. In fact, the irony is, we need it. Yes. Inflammation promotes a healthy body – in small amounts. Suffice it to say, without inflammation, we would not be alive.

Chapter 8. Ketosis is Anti-Inflammatory

What Is Inflammation?

There are three types of inflammation: (1) acute inflammation, (2) silent inflammation, and (3) fat cell inflammation or what Dr. Lori refers to as *FatFlammation.* In fact, Dr. Lori wrote an entire book called *How to Fight FATFlammation*, and if you want more detail about the concepts she lays out in this chapter, we'd highly encourage you to read it. Inflammation plays such a huge role in disease and health that anyone who wants to improve their health should learn as much as they can about it! But for now, let's go over the "Cliff's Notes" version.

Every one of us is acutely aware of inflammation. How do we know this? Because we experience it frequently. Every time you have been injured or sick, such as with a terrible head cold, a sprained ankle, a painful sunburn, or a cut on the finger, *acute inflammation* (and it's not so "cute") comes rushing to the rescue. You may think that the pain, swelling, and tenderness of a sprained ankle is not a good thing – well, actually it is.

Without acute inflammation, we simply would cease to exist. This type of inflammation is an immune response that protects us, keeps us alive, and keeps us healthy. Without it, we would be in big trouble.

Let's take that cut on the finger. When you cut your finger, an enormous amount of inflammatory molecules are released and "soldiers" if you will, rush to the site to repair the wound. These soldiers repair the wound, and then go away, then the inflammation goes away, and all is well.

However, when acute inflammation doesn't heal, but instead continues to spew out inflammatory compounds that the soldiers can't keep up with, it becomes chronic or silent inflammation. This continual process is the core cause of most illness, disease, faster aging, and weight gain. This chronic, or silent inflammation is the type of inflammation we do not want. This type of damaging inflammation is there 24/7, lurking...unbeknownst to you. In fact, 75% of all Americans are walking around with this damaging, low-level inflammation and are not even aware of it.

You can look at silent inflammation as like having a sore on the inside of your body that never heals – it's always there. Its very silence at the outset is the issue.

Ketosis and Inflammation

How does the ketosis factor into this? Well, silent inflammation specifically, triggers something called the NLRP3 inflammasome – an immune system receptor that triggers the secretion of potent pro-inflammatory molecules called cytokines, which factor into the start or progression of diseases with a high impact on our health, such as metabolic disorders and neurodegenerative diseases.

This is where ketosis, and more specifically, the ketone *beta-hydroxybutyrate* (BHB) comes into play. BHB has been shown to block this pesky inflammasome and thereby inhibit the development of NLRP3 related inflammatory diseases. By triggering ketosis and production of the ketone BHB, we may be able to help reduce how much the NLRP3 inflammasome fires in the body. This is also a reason that people are looking at the potential for ketone supplementation – to boost levels of BHB in the body.

BHB and other ketones also mitigate inflammation (including brain inflammation) by a protein that is activated in the presence of BHB called CTBP or C-terminal binding protein. This protein actually modulates a specific genetic response to inflammation, so it's not just temporarily taking away inflammation like an aspirin or ibuprofen would do, it is actually changing a little bit of your genetic code to make it less likely that you will have inflammation occurring overall.

"Silent inflammation is the core underlying cause of most illness, disease, faster-aging and weight gain." – Dr. Lori Shemek, "How to Fight FATflammation"

Whatever you call it, silent, chronic or low-level, this type of persistent inflammation is unlike acute inflammation because it is imperceptible – it is below the perception of pain. That's one of the reasons it's referred to as "silent" inflammation, because it's quiet – rather than being noticeable like painful acute inflammation. And unlike acute inflammation, silent inflammation emits just a constant trickle of inflammatory molecules, which causes damage to your body over time. In addition, one of the things chronic inflammation does is disrupt hormonal signaling at the cellular level, and that leads to increased fat accumulation, acceleration in the development of chronic diseases, and decreased physical performance.

Multiple diseases such as cancer, stroke, Alzheimer's disease, diabetes, and obesity, high blood pressure, rheumatoid arthritis, heart disease and many more, are all directly linked to this low-level cellular inflammation.

Many people living with these diseases where inflammation is the underlying cause are looking for treatment or therapy. Unfortunately, there isn't currently any medication one can take to kick inflammation to the curb without repercussions or side effects. We all know that anti-inflammatory drugs can take away the inflammation and pain for a period of time. The problem is that these drugs, including over the counter medications like ibuprofen, all work on a different biochemical pathway in the body, and can leave us with side effects, and in many cases, secondary health issues.

This is where ketosis and the **ketogenic diet** are beneficial – they can help heal, reduce, prevent and even reverse inflammation, and without the side effects of medications. Living a long, active life largely depends on the health and well being of your cellular health and ultimately your mitochondrial health, which is what being in a state of ketosis will accomplish.

"A powerful tool to combat inflammation comes not from the pharmacy, but from the grocery store." ~Dr. Mark Hyman, author of *Eat Fat, Get Thin*

How can you hit the inflammatory rewind button and reprogram your genes to a fat-burning and inflammation-free state? By making different choices starting today. Let's talk about some of the causes of inflammation so that we can begin to identify better dietary and lifestyle changes to keep inflammation at bay!

What Are The Main Causes of Inflammation?

The main drivers of low-level, silent inflammation that wreaks havoc with our health and quality of life include the following:

Sugar

When you ingest simple carbohydrates (such as sugar, sucrose, or fructose), white flour or refined flour products (such as pasta, bagels, breads, crackers or chips), whole wheat products, fruit juices and the like, the body very quickly breaks the carbohydrates within these foods down into sugars that are rapidly infused into our blood, and our blood glucose levels are elevated. Then the hormone insulin is released to shuttle that glucose out of the blood so it can be used or stored. With a constant intake of high-sugar and high carbohydrate foods, glucose remains elevated, and insulin levels also spike, leading to inflammation. If the inflammation is chronic (constant or long-term) – which is the case when people eat multiple meals and snacks a day consisting of these sorts of high-sugar and high carbohydrate foods – it can lead to metabolic diseases such as obesity, type 2 diabetes, cardiovascular disease, and more.

Standard American Diet

Related to sugar is the Standard American Diet (SAD). SAD is an excellent example of the main dietary drivers of inflammation because it is mostly a diet of convenience – with its foods mostly containing highly processed and refined carbohydrates, large amount of processed seed oils, copious amounts of obvious, added and hidden sugars, and only a small amount of vegetables and other natural nutrient-dense foods.

There is an antiquated notion that we, as humans, require carbohydrates for optimal health. The truth is, fat is the preferred fuel of human metabolism and has been for most of human evolution. Under normal human circumstances, we actually require only minimal amounts of glucose. Yet, the Standard American Diet is typically anywhere from 60-80% carbohydrates, and those carbs chronically raise blood glucose, which in turn causes silent inflammation. This constant, excess intake of carbohydrates has created an inflamed, fat and sick society.

Omega 6 Fat

Omega 6 fat is necessary for our health as it is an essential fat – and we can only get it through our diet. However, food manufacturers have found a way to process omega oils that harm us on a cellular level, such as canola oil and vegetable oils. These oils create an imbalance between two essential fats – omega 6 and omega 3, and impede our ability to fight inflammation.

Now, omega 3 oil's main role is to tamp down inflammation, but often it cannot accomplish this role because the majority of individuals are ingesting an excess of omega 6 fats (from the aforementioned processed vegetable oils) preventing any anti-inflammatory effect by the omega 3 oils. Additionally, an excess amount of omega 6 fat not only promotes inflammation, but also promotes the compound arachidonic acid. Arachidonic acid is somewhat controversial because it has both health-promoting and health-eroding qualities, but has been associated with fat storage and inflammation. The bottom line is that it's important that we avoid processed omega 6 oils and get the right amount of them naturally along with some omega 3 oils.

Excess Weight and Obesity

Another cause of inflammation is the excess weight (fat) most individuals are carrying around now. In fact, 70% of most Americans are overweight or obese – a staggering statistic. The present expert consensus on the effects of excess weight is that it increases the incidence of nearly all age-related disease, shortens life expectancy, and raises overall lifetime medical expenditure primarily due to the raised levels of chronic inflammation produced by fat tissue. In fact, researchers forecast close to *half* the United States population will be obese and one-quarter will have severe obesity by 2030.

The book *How to Fight FATflammation*, takes a deep dive into fat cell inflammation and its causative and persistent cyclical role in weight gain (we encourage you to read it to get a more in-depth explanation on this crucial aspect of health).

We all have roughly 100 million fat cells (adipocytes) in our body and they are about the size of a period on the end of sentence. With the types of foods we are ingesting such as refined, processed, nutrient void, high calorie and dense carbohydrate foods, we are packing our fat cells with glucose, fat and other compounds. The fat cell then becomes more and more bloated, leading to a vicious cycle of fat cell inflammation. This silent inflammation is releasing inflammatory molecules 24/7. The more fat that is stored in the fat cells, the more of these inflammatory molecules are released and thus, the relentless cycle of more and more inflammation and weight gain.

When insulin levels go up — say, after a meal — fat cells take in more fatty acids, literally swelling in size. When insulin levels drop, fat cells release their stores as a source of energy for the body. This process is exactly where ketosis and the ketogenic diet can come into play. You see, because the ketogenic diet is very low in carbohydrates, it keeps blood glucose stable, and therefore the body doesn't need to release insulin to counteract the blood glucose levels. The ketogenic diet can help coax your fat cells into releasing those stores of fatty acids, as well as quell their release of inflammatory molecules.

Fat is more than just unsightly and inconvenient – it's linked to a number of different diseases and comorbid conditions. The most inflammatory fat on our body is good old belly fat, also called visceral fat. This type of fat has been linked with inflammatory conditions (such as insulin resistance, metabolic syndrome, heart disease, high blood pressure, hormone balance upset, and type 2 diabetes), to an increased risk for certain cancers, and contributes to the cycle of fat gain and elevated inflammatory molecule release. Visceral fat is deep-seated in your body, and surrounds the organs and muscles in your chest, stomach and abdomen. Again, where the ketogenic diet comes in, is that it helps coax your body into using that visceral fat as fuel, instead of storing it and impacting your organs.

Aging

Aging is defined as the progressive accumulation of damage over time, leading to disturbed function on the cellular, tissue and organ level, and eventually leading to disease and death.

There are multiple theories being researched on the aging process. There is a branch of aging related research called *"Inflamm-Aging."* Increasingly, evidence indicates that inflamm-aging (inflammation) is intensively associated with many aging diseases, such as Alzheimer's disease, atherosclerosis and heart disease,

Chapter 8. Ketosis is Anti-Inflammatory

type II diabetes, and cancer, although the exact mechanisms involved are not completely understood. We do know that inflammation plays a huge role in aging and accelerated aging. When inflammation is constant, regeneration and tissue maintenance begin to decline, cancer rates rise, and many disease processes accelerate.

When we are young, with our accompanying youthful cells that have healthy and plentiful mitochondria, incidental unhealthy food choices, such as multiple bowls of ice cream, do not make much of a negative health impact. But as we age, these unhealthy choices make a bigger and bigger impact because our body is not able to counteract the damage on a cellular level as easily.

Fortunately for us, ketosis can slow the aging process. Many of the 300 purported theories of aging, such as the Free Radical Theory of Aging or the Glycation Theory of Aging, are mitigated with ketosis or ketone bodies. Ketone bodies act as antioxidants and anti-inflammatory agents that also provide benefit and potential reversal of several neurological disorders in which oxidative stress at the cellular level is strongly implicated as a cause. These disorders include Alzheimer's disease, ALS, traumatic brain injury, Parkinson's disease, and stroke. Not surprisingly, these are diseases that we see increased incidence of as people age.

The Free Radical Theory of Aging: free radicals, which are chemically reactive molecules (sometimes called Reactive Oxygen Species, or ROS), can bind to our cells, causing damage and inflammation to our DNA and other proteins in our body. Keto, as we've mentioned, helps to reduce systemic inflammation at the cellular level.

The Glycation Theory of Aging: Glycation or Advanced Glycation End-Products (AGES) is the process whereby circulating sugars in the blood attach to proteins, changing the nature and structure of all tissues in our body (including our skin), leading to faster aging. Glycation rises as sugars in the blood increase. So back to what we've discussed previously, it's imperative that we control blood sugar levels, and the ketosis does this very effectively.

In general, low carb diets, and especially the ketogenic diet, improve blood sugar control and reduce hunger, as they mimic the effects of fasting. Research has also shown that reduced calorie consumption decreases oxidative damage within the body.

Along with reducing oxidative damage, ketosis also helps to promote healthy mitochondria, the power plants of your cells, by increasing mitochondrial glutathione. Glutathione is called the "mother of all antioxidants." Many people try to take supplemental glutathione, but it is not that bio-available or readily absorbed when taken orally. However, ketosis, and specifically ketone bodies such as BHB, influence this organelle directly and provide benefits. Remember, poor mitochondrial health and inflammation go hand-in-hand.

Keto has another important benefit for health and inflammation: it can also reduce triglycerides, which are fatty acids in the blood stream. Elevated triglycerides are markers for increased heart disease risk and inflammation.

The fundamental take-away is that reducing your blood sugar also reduces blood insulin levels, glycation, and inflammation, and this equates to optimal health. Because ketosis helps with all these aspects, it's showing to be a very effective tool in the fight against age-related inflammation.

Unhealthy Gut Bacteria

The importance of our gut health cannot be overstated: our gut houses 70% of our immune system, and our mental health is connected to it as well. It is estimated that 90% of the feel-good neurotransmitter *serotonin (we call it the "happy transmitter") is* made in the gut and not in the brain as was previously thought. New research suggests that we have 500 million brain cells in the lining of our gut, so our gut is considered our "second brain." Even our weight is directly impacted by our gut microflora. So you can sense how crucial it is to ensure we create and maintain a healthy gut microbiome.

We have 40 trillion gut bacteria and that equates to roughly 3-5 pounds of these little critters that we are walking around with. Unfortunately, the majority of people have an abundance of unhealthy gut microbes and a poor number of diverse species because of their poor dietary choices.

With the typical diet, individuals are unknowingly feeding their unhealthy microbes with the very foods these unhealthy critters need to survive: sugar, refined and processed foods, few vegetables, and excess carbohydrates – in other words, the Standard American Diet (SAD, both literally and figuratively!). These unhealthy foods are necessary for the survival and abundance of specific types of gut bacteria that promote inflammation and more.

We need to create a healthy gut foundation. A healthy gut has two basic "musts" – **prebiotics and probiotics**. Prebiotics are plant-fiber compounds and what we refer to as *fertilizer* for the healthy bacteria – they feed these important microbes to help facilitate optimal health and weight loss. Probiotics have the same end-result, but instead of feeding the bacteria, they *are* the good healthy bacteria that are planted within the gut. You can find these probiotics from delicious cultured and fermented foods such as yogurt, kefir, sauerkraut, olives, pickles and many others. When prebiotics and probiotics are combined, they create a *powerful* healthful effect.

We can begin to take control of our health by feeding our microbiome with the right foods. Essentially, what we eat (or choose not to eat) determines the type of bacteria we grow in our gut garden. The healthier the balance of gut bacteria, by correcting the imbalance or overgrowth of unhealthy gut bacteria, the more likely it is that you will lose weight, create optimal health and improve mental well-being. This is where the ketogenic diet comes in!

The ketogenic diet provides the gut with prebiotics, which provide the nutrition for probiotics. The keto diet is helpful at starving the harmful bacteria found in the gut (including small intestinal bacterial overgrowth), and allowing the healthy good bacteria thrive. It also helps in maintaining a healthy gut lining, and appears to play a role in healing leaky gut syndrome.

Sedentary Lifestyle

We all know that exercise and staying mostly active promotes good health. But what about the reverse? An abundance of robust research shows that lack of movement in our lives leads to inflammation and its resulting negative health conditions.

Let's take simply sitting. The longer we sit, the more of an increase we have in inflammatory bio-markers such as c-reactive protein (particularly in men), chronic low-grade inflammation, insulin resistance, and weight gain, particularly belly fat.

The key takeaway is that to prevent inflammation that leads to chronic disease, we need to spend less time sitting. Get up and move! Ketones provide natural energy, which improves the motivation to move more, which is yet another way the ketogenic diet or exogenous ketone supplementation can help!

Nutrient Deficiencies

Nutrient deficiencies are an extremely common cause of inflammation for the majority of people eating the standard American diet, because the majority of food intake is void of nutrients and full of inflammatory compounds. This can be corrected with the ketogenic diet and other lifestyle choices.

These are the top nutrient deficiencies according to various research sources:
.
Omega-3
Vitamin D
B Vitamins (Particularly B-6 and B-12)
Selenium
Zinc
Magnesium
Potassium
Iodine

Foods to Eat to Reduce Inflammation

Inflammation can occur from various causes, but what may surprise you is that a significant source of chronic inflammation is the food that we eat. The great thing about the ketogenic diet is that keto-friendly foods (and ketones themselves) also tend to be anti-inflammatory!

Here is a list of top ketogenic AND anti-inflammatory foods that help the body fight inflammation:

- **Healthy fats** like egg yolks (preferably pasture-raised); healthy oils like coconut oil, olive oil, MCT oil or powder, and avocado oil; nuts and seeds; fatty fish like shellfish, salmon, and sardines; avocados; and butters such as grass-fed butter or ghee, coconut butter, and cocoa butter.
- **Omega-3 fats** are especially important for fighting inflammation. Make sure you get them from omega-3-rich eggs, wild or cold-water fish, or an omega-3 supplement if necessary.
- **Healthy meats** that are grass-fed (also contain omega-3 fat), and pastured-raised fatty versions. Good options are bison, beef, organ meats, lamb, pork, and fatty fish.
- **Non-starchy vegetables** like dark leafy greens: spinach, chard, collards, kale, cauliflower, and broccoli.

Inflammatory Foods to Avoid

Stay away from foods that are high in sugars or processed ingredients. Of course, these are things you cannot eat if you are trying to achieve ketosis, but it's good to read through and know this list anyway. Specifically, here are some of the <u>main things to avoid</u> regardless of whether you are going full keto, using ketone supplements, or simply trying to reduce inflammation in your body:

- **Processed foods that are packaged and refined.** That includes soy "vegan" products, condiments, and frozen meals. Basically if it's fast food or pre-prepared frozen food, it is likely highly processed and therefore promotes the silent inflammation we've described.
- **High-glycemic foods** such as all sugars, grains (yes, even whole grains), fruits, and starchy vegetables. Glycemic means that it converts quickly to sugar in your blood stream, which as we know, causes insulin release, and its subsequent inflammation.
- **Refined vegetable and seed oils,** especially those high in inflammatory omega 6 fat such as canola oil, corn, vegetable, and soybean oils
- **Juices, sodas and energy drinks.** Stick with water, coffee or herbal tea. Fruit juices are just liquid sugar. Even though we've been told our whole lives that a big glass of orange juice is good

for us, the fact is, it's a big glass of fructose, which is a form of sugar, and it impacts our body the same way as any other sugar. There are better sources of vitamin C and anti-oxidants then fruit juices. Sodas, even sugar free or diet sodas, contain a plethora of inflammatory chemicals including artificial sweeteners. And most energy drinks are full of the same types of chemicals and additives.

The bottom line is that keto supplements and the ketogenic diet can act as an excellent, natural way to promote an anti-inflammatory state in our bodies.

Sleep

Lacking sleep? Many people are lacking this vital recurring state, and it is worth noting that a lack of sleep is inflammatory. Lack of sleep increases stress hormones (see below) and reduces the amount of time our body has to heal itself, and leads to silent inflammation. So getting plenty of sleep is a key part of reducing chronic, low-level inflammation.

Stress

When we are under psychological stress — such as when we feel challenged or threatened — the body releases stress hormones such as epinephrine and norepinephrine as part of the classic "fight-or-flight" response. This is not necessarily bad. We needed those stress hormones to escape from that saber-toothed tiger eons ago, and we probably experience them now when it's time to give a speech or other activities that raise our stress levels!

Stress hormones also stimulate the production of pro-inflammatory signaling molecules, and when stress hormone release is constant, or chronic, it can cause inflammation that creates a cascade of bio-chemical reactions leading to weight gain, poor health, and lack of sleep, which by the way, create a vicious cycle amongst themselves.

It is when our stress response becomes an every day experience or feeling, this is then what we call chronic stress.

Chronic stress can also wreak havoc with the hormone cortisol, which helps control the inflammatory response. When left unchecked, weight gain and anxiety can occur from unbalanced cortisol levels.

Once again, ketones to the rescue! The ketogenic diet, and more specifically, the ketone bodies created by the ketogenic diet, intermittent fasting, exercise or taken as therapeutic supplements, have been shown to reduce the stress, anxiety and anxiety-related disorders that impede not just our quality life, but our health as well. Researchers are now assessing therapeutic ketone supplements and the ketogenic diet as potential treatments or therapy for certain psychological disorders, including depression and anxiety, which is great news for many who suffer from them. It is becoming more and more clear that diet, supplementation, and nutrition play a key role in helping us overcome, and even prevent, many diverse neurologic disorders, especially when inflammation is at their core.

Summary

In summary, inflammation can cause significant damage to our health. Getting into ketosis through diet, fasting, ketone supplementation, and exercise, is key! The ketogenic diet helps coax the body to produce the anti-inflammatory ketone beta-hydroxybutyrate (BHB). Intermittent fasting, exercise and supplementing with exogenous BHB can also help mitigate inflammatory processes. And the foods that make up the ketogenic diet tend to quell inflammation. So for all these reasons, ketosis is the key to beating inflammation and optimizing your health!

Chapter 9. Keto and Auto-Immune Diseases, Multiple Sclerosis and Polycystic Ovary Syndrome (PCOS)

How is life with autoimmune disease? It can be challenging, scary and yet, surprisingly and ironically, it is the side effect of a robust immune system.

Those who have autoimmune disease know only too well how the daily fight can be. Autoimmune disease is a type of immune 'dysfunction' – a condition arising from an abnormal or heightened immune response to a normal body part.

There are at least 80 types of autoimmune diseases, which is a staggering statistic. They include diseases such as: Hashimoto's thyroid disease, multiple sclerosis, autoimmune hepatitis, lupus, rheumatoid arthritis, psoriasis, Addison's disease, Grave's disease and many more. Nearly any body part can be involved, and common symptoms include low-grade fever, pain, skin disorders, and fatigue. For people who have autoimmune disease, the most menial daily things can be incredibly challenging, exhausting, and painful.

What is a day in the life of a person with the autoimmune condition Hashimoto's disease? It's a day that is a constant struggle for most. They struggle with fatigue, and so they must follow a very clean diet, ensure they are getting enough sleep, and even with better sleep and diet, they often still have brain fog. They are very aware that chronic stress (which can add stress itself) can cause flare-ups causing more symptoms such as thinning hair, back pain, joint pain, dry skin, and exhaustion. Imagine dealing with all of this! And yet there's more. Those with autoimmune disease such as Hashimoto's can suffer mental health disorders such as depression and anxiety. In short, chronic illness is a daily thing for people with autoimmune disorders, and some suffer with more than just one condition.

Chapter 10: Keto and Respiratory Diseases

With an autoimmune disease, the body becomes inflamed and stays inflamed because it can't heal and function, because your immune system is attacking itself. The body is creating antibodies, which means *"against the body"* – in essence, against its own tissue. It is essentially a self-attack because the body, in a sense, is having an allergy to its own tissues.

Multiple Sclerosis

Once again, there is hope, thanks to ketogenic therapies. Research shows that the ketogenic diet has led to very positive outcomes in some people with multiple sclerosis. They have experienced reversal of symptoms and remyelination where other dietary interventions have not been successful. Research is also showing that following a ketogenic diet long term is safe, feasible, and potentially effective in the treatment of multiple sclerosis (RRMS) patients.

Terry Wahls, MD, a physician and professor at the University of Iowa and author of the Wahls Protocol (https://terrywahls.com/), is an excellent example of someone who took her multiple sclerosis into her own hands. Her remarkable story serves as validation that when we start with our diet, we can make powerful changes.

Dr. Wahls says that she had transitioned from primary MS to secondary progressive multiple sclerosis, and underwent chemotherapy in an attempt to slow the disease. She also began using a tilt-recline wheelchair because of weakness in her back muscles. At this point, she had resigned herself to eventually becoming bedridden due to the disease's ravages — an outcome she wanted to forestall for as long as possible.

Yet, she actually healed her condition! How did Dr. Wahls heal her autoimmune disease? She first adopted the nutrient-rich paleo diet, gradually refining it to a ketogenic diet/paleo diet combined with intermittent fasting to help heal her autoimmune disease. She was able to stop using her wheelchair and is now walking and biking and no longer sitting in a wheelchair, and her MS is in remission – she is living a full and healthy life. Her entire story is recounted on her website noted above. The bottom line is that the ketogenic diet has excellent potential to help people with MS and with other autoimmune diseases.

The Power of Fat

Part of the success of the ketogenic diet is in the breakdown of the macros. Fat is a key player! The large percentage of fat in the ketogenic diet is very nurturing for the nervous system and the immune system, as well as helping to regulate hormones. In fact, before antibiotics, physicians would give patients with tuberculosis a cup of raw cream mixed with egg yolk because they knew, way back then, that cholesterol improves immune function. You can then imagine how well the immune system would function with a diet that contains these types of foods.

The ketogenic diet can include organ meats such as liver and heart. Many people are unaware that not just meats, but organ meats in particular, are potent sources of nutrients and have more vitamins and minerals than many fruits or vegetables. You will find more vitamin C and potassium (very common deficiencies in those with autoimmune diseases) including vitamin A, E and D in organ meats vs plants, and that is why those with autoimmune issues or other health conditions respond so well on this diet.

The ketogenic diet as well as ketone supplementation can markedly reduce or reverse inflammation and optimize the immune response. This could make the ketosis an effective tool for reversing the symptoms of autoimmunity, and is well worth trying for those suffering from one of these debilitating syndromes or diseases.

Polycystic Ovary Syndrome

Polycystic Ovary Syndrome (PCOS) is the most common endocrine disorder among pre-menopausal women. Even though you may have never heard of it, is a very common health condition affecting millions of women. As its name implies, the syndrome often results in women having multiple fluid-filled cysts in their ovaries; however, not all women with PCOS have the cysts.

Chapter 10: Keto and Respiratory Diseases

As we've shown throughout this book, an increasing amount of recent evidence has accumulated in the literature, suggesting that very-low-carbohydrate ketogenic diets, as well as ketone supplements, can have a therapeutic role in numerous diseases, and that includes PCOS.

What are the Key Hallmarks of PCOS?

PCOS is a multi-symptom and multi-factorial syndrome, in other words, there are a number of causes, contributors, and symptoms, and not all women who have PCOS have all the same symptoms and triggers. Although it is considered a hormonal issue (often associated with excess androgens and insulin), the exact cause is not known. But the main hallmarks of PCOS include heart disease, blood lipid abnormalities, obesity, type 2 diabetes, missed menstrual cycles or major menstrual irregularities, fatigue, hair growth in unexpected places (chest, stomach, thighs, chin and more), thinning or balding of the head, acne, unexplained persistent weight gain, insulin resistance, skin tags appearing around the neck and under the arms, infertility (difficulty getting pregnant), and more. It's worth noting that PCOS is seen more frequently in obese patients, and obesity is believed to be either causative or symptomatic – and perhaps both. It also is most common of women in their reproductive years, so although it's often seen in young women, older women who are still fertile can have it too.

What is also important to note is that because its cause is not completely understood, the medical establishment has treated PCOS only to manage the symptoms, without curing the underlying cause of this terrible condition.

But before you become frustrated with the medical experts, there is some very promising news! Scientists and researchers have found that very low-carb nutrition, such as the ketogenic diet, can have a marked effect in alleviating and reversing the symptoms and even healing PCOS. Some evidence has suggested that a diet with a higher ratio of protein to carbohydrates has metabolic advantages in the treatment of polycystic ovary syndrome (PCOS).

In women that participated in a 2005 study using the ketogenic diet for weight loss, "there were significant reductions from baseline to 24 weeks in body weight (-12%), percent free testosterone (-22%), LH/FSH ratio (-36%), and fasting insulin (-54%). Furthermore, two of those women became pregnant despite previous infertility problems."

In fact, research shows that the ketogenic diet can reverse symptoms and promote weight loss and increase lean body mass for those with PCOS in as little as 8 weeks, and which, over time, may improve reproductive/endocrine outcomes. This makes complete sense when you examine the ketogenic diet independent of its effects upon overall health, such as increasing insulin sensitivity, promoting weight loss, balancing hormones, reversing inflammation, healing acne, and more.

Do We Know What Causes PCOS?

The answer is an absolute, definite "sort of." Researchers believe that genetics play a role, hormone imbalances are a driver, and environmental exposures have an impact as well. Beyond that, though, it's still pretty murky. And with a condition so common, PCOS is baffling because researchers have not yet determined an exact cause or reason why some have it and others don't develop it, and why it presents so differently in different women.

However, an intriguing recent study has possibly brought us closer to an understanding of a potential cause: exposure to high levels of a hormone called anti-Müllerian while in the womb. However, it is preliminary research in animals, and not yet studied in humans, so the jury is not out on this quite yet.

In terms of genetics, researchers propose that there are specific genetic variants that contribute to PCOS. For example, a recent study by Miller and colleagues concluded that we might be able to explain the association of PCOS and insulin resistance by a single genetic defect.

Regardless of the exact cause, insulin is a key player in this disease. In women with PCOS, up to 80% are insulin-resistant, which means they have higher levels of circulating insulin in their system. The hormone insulin facilitates excess androgen production directly and indirectly in women with PCOS, and those androgens can cause increasing symptoms such as acne, insulin resistance, mood swings, high blood pressure, and excessive facial and body hair growth.

Additionally, insulin also keeps at bay a key circulating protein that binds to testosterone and, thus, increases circulating testosterone that has a great impact upon the previously mentioned androgenic symptoms.

PCOS cannot be diagnosed by symptoms alone. For example, there are many women with high testosterone, for example, that do not have this condition. Therefore, in order to confirm a PCOS diagnosis, it's recommended to order blood tests to measure hormone levels, an ultrasound to look at reproductive organs, and thorough personal and family history (as there is a genetic component).

Despite no known cause, we do know that the ketogenic diet and ketone supplementation have been reported to help alleviate (and in some cases reverse) the symptoms for many, and improve fertility outcomes.

How Does the Ketogenic Diet and Being in Ketosis Help PCOS?

Research shows a clear association between PCOS and high carbohydrate foods, excess calorie consumption, inactivity, increased insulin levels and insulin resistance, and higher body fat levels. It then stands to reason that markedly reducing carbohydrates and increasing fat consumption to achieve ketosis (as we have discussed in the previous chapters) will in turn lower and stabilize blood glucose, reduce insulin levels and eventually increase insulin sensitivity, encourage the body to begin using body fat for fuel (leading to a reduction in fat storage and body fat mass), and will help balance hormones. This all helps lead to other outcomes such as weight loss, restored menstrual cycles, restored fertility, improved cardiovascular health, less acne, and much more.

In short, ketosis addresses many of the root causes and contributors of PCOS, and should be considered as a potential therapy by women who suffer from the symptoms of PCOS. The Ketogenic Key lifestyle addresses and treats many of the core underlying causes thought to be responsible for PCOS, and isn't that the ultimate prescription for health?

Chapter 10: Keto and Respiratory Diseases

Another one of the exciting areas of emerging research for ketone therapeutics is lung disease. There are four key areas of interest in how ketones and ketogenic nutrition impact the lungs. First, the ketogenic diet and the ketone body beta-hydroxybutyrate have been shown to be anti-inflammatory. Second, the ketogenic diet has been shown to support numerous molecules and signalers that fight oxidative stress and reactive oxygen species. Third, a high-fat diet has been shown to improve gas exchange and reduce CO_2 production. And fourth, glucose homeostasis (specifically lower glucose levels) has been shown to have a positive impact on lung disease such as COPD and lung infections that accompany or result from various lung conditions.

Although heart disease and cancer get most of the attention for fatalities, lung disease deaths are alarmingly high. Chronic obstructive pulmonary disease (COPD) is one of the most prevalent and deadly diseases in the world, currently the 4th leading cause of death worldwide and projected to move to 3rd very soon. It is a progressive disease that has no cure and requires management as it progresses over time. It is characterized by a combination of obstructive lung disease, chronic emphysema, and potential frequent acute or chronic infections such as bronchitis and pneumonia. Chances are, you know someone who has COPD.

It is increasingly being realized that nutrition may be able to play a significant role in helping to alleviate the inflammation and other underlying aspects of the disease that affect its severity. The fact that a high-fat diet helps improve gas exchange in the lungs is not a new concept. Researchers have known that high-fat nutrition is useful in hospitalized COPD patients. However, only recently have they begun to recognize that a high-fat (low-carb) diet in non-hospitalized patients might be useful!

In 2019, a review of data from the National Health and Nutrition Examination Surveys (NHANES) looked at the relationship between saturated fat intake and lung function, and found increased lung function associated with increased saturated fat intake in patients with COPD.

An outstanding 2013 literature review in the *European Journal of Clinical Nutrition* noted the following about the usefulness of the ketogenic diet in respiratory disorders:
"The metabolic effects of a ketogenic diet imply a higher-than-usual oxidation of fats, which leads in turn to reduced respiratory exchange ratio values...." "Hence, following a ketogenic diet-induced decrement of the respiratory exchange ratio and of metabolic carbon dioxide output, a decrease in arterial carbon dioxide partial pressure or of pulmonary ventilation, or of both, is expected. **If verified, these effects might be useful in the treatment of patients with respiratory failure;** however, this aspect of the ketogenic diet remains to be investigated."

Anecdotal evidence from patients indicates that a high-fat, low carb diet can help improve symptoms of COPD. Some researchers believe that this may be because COPD is a disease marked by underlying inflammation of the airways, and is NLRP3 inflammasome mediated. As we know, the ketone body beta-hydroxybutyrate has been shown to inhibit NLRP3 mediated inflammation. To our knowledge, no studies to date have specifically looked at ketone supplementation or a ketogenic diet intervention in COPD patients, although we are aware of some case studies with individual patients currently being prepared for publication.

Another potential therapeutic action of the ketogenic diet is upregulation of glutathione, a vital intra- and extracellular antioxidant in the lungs. Studies have shown that the ketogenic diet increases glutathione levels, as well as nrf2 levels (a cellular signaler of anti-oxidant activity). So in addition to potential inhibition of NLRP3 inflammation, it appears that ketone bodies also support signaling of antioxidants that protect lung epithelium, especially in models of COPD and emphysema and other types of inflammatory lung disease and lung injury.

Chapter 11. Keto and Migraines

An emerging area of focus is glucose homeostasis (stability of glucose levels) as well as the glucose concentrations of airway surface liquid (ASL) in the lungs. Research shows that high glucose levels in ASL allows certain types of bacteria to proliferate more easily, whereas lower glucose ASL levels appear to inhibit bacterial growth. Therefore, researchers are calling for research into glucose lowering drugs to see if they can have an impact. Sadly, they haven't yet made the connection to controlling

Nutritional supplements with a high-calorie, high-fat content have been recommended in the cases of malnourished COPD patients, but current global COPD guidelines do not make any recommendations for ongoing nutrition or sustained dietary changes, most likely due to the lack of reliable evidence from studies in patients. The need for more research on the ketogenic diet and ketone supplementation in lung diseases like COPD is very evident, and we hope that the points we make will spur patients to discuss options with their physicians and prompt clinicians and researchers to do more than simply treat hospitalized and malnourished patients with supplementation. This is an area of therapy that bears watching and speaking out about.

At the time of this writing, there is very little offered in terms of nutritional guidelines as part of ongoing COPD management and therapy or in the fight against inflammatory lung diseases and lung infections, yet there is scientific evidence that these interventions may help.

Chapter 11. Keto and Migraines

What is a migraine? Before you think it is a type of a headache, let me tell you, it is not "just a headache." It's still controversial in the scientific arena whether a migraine is primarily vascular (involving blood vessels) or a neurological dysfunction (involving neurons and the nervous system and brain), but it's likely that both have a significant role to play. What we do know is that the core underlying cause is probably inflammation.

Living with migraines is a nightmare for so many. Here is an excerpt from *The Mighty – A Day in the Life of a Person with Migraine:*

> *"Imagine a scenario when you wake up with a crane lifting you off the bed with your head mounted on the hook. Then think of walking to work with an iron ball tied to each of your ankles. Visualize sitting in front of a screen that recklessly shoots light bullets into your eye for at least eight hours a day. Your head pounds at breakneck speed, making you dizzy as you walk back home, now with four iron balls tied to your head. Wait, wait, wait... did you think this is all? No, it doesn't end here.*
>
> *Towards twilight you are almost like a zombie. You get back home energy-less, irked, tired, jaded, only wanting to get into your "Palace of Darkness" where silence, darkness and concealment wait for you. So you miss the beautiful sunrise, you miss fun at work, you miss enjoying life with your family, you miss screaming when your favorite team wins a game, you miss dancing to your favorite song, you miss being happy or sad without having to worry about a "hangover" headache... You miss life, because your life is here with you all the time, your migraine."*

Migraines are a disorder that is characterized by hyper-excitable brain networks that may be triggered by a variety of stimuli (*e.g.* alcohol, menstruation, fragrances, light glare), or even during sleep, leading to severe migraine attacks. Thirty-six million Americans, about 12% of the population, suffer from migraine headaches. Migraines are three times more common in women than men. Migraines will affect 30% of women at some point during their lifetime.

During a migraine attack, the sufferer may experience auras, which in many cases act as a warning sign a migraine is impending. Once it does occur, the migraine sufferer may see flashing or shimmering lights, zigzagging lines, or stars. Some people describe psychedelic types of images. It may also cause blind spots in the field of vision. The migraine can also cause debilitating head pain, nausea, vomiting, and sensitivity to smells, noise and light, leading the migraine sufferer to do almost anything to ward off an attack.

"One of the reasons migraine is so common is because so many pathways lead to migraine," says Richard Lipton, MD, director of the Montefiore Headache Center in New York City, "and those pathways may differ from person to person."

That can make treating migraines more difficult; what works for one person might not work for another.

Ketogenic Diet and Migraines

Many people take prescription or over the counter drugs to ward off an attack. This may work well for some but not for others. Therefore, many people are at a loss as to what to do to help this painful condition. As you may have guessed by now, this is where the ketogenic diet and ketone bodies can help. The ketogenic diet has been shown to mitigate or prevent the occurrence, to reduce the frequency and severity of these attacks.

Can simply eating a diet high in fat, very low in carbohydrates and moderate protein really have a powerful impact upon migraines? Dr. Josh Turnkett, neurologist and author of *The Migraine Miracle* thinks so and states:

> "We've only just begun to see glimpses of the therapeutic potential of ketogenic diets beyond the treatment of epilepsy, including cancer, neurodegenerative disorders (Alzheimer's, Parkinson's, etc.), obesity, and migraine."

Research published in the European Journal of Neurology showed that 96 women following a ketogenic diet had significant decreases in the number of days with headaches and pain relief medication in a short period of time.

It is thought that the underlying mechanisms of the ketogenic diet's positive impact could be related in its ability to enhance mitochondrial energy metabolism in the brain, and counteract neural inflammation.

Migraine organizations such as the American Migraine Foundation are targeting glutamate as a serious perpetrator in those with migraines. **Although food-related migraine triggers vary by person, one of the most-often cited triggers is monosodium glutamate or MSG. The trouble is, it's in so many foods and comes under so many aliases that it's hard to keep it out of our diets.** Foods that contain significant amounts of glutamic acid or glutamate (different chemicals but extremely similar in their effect on promoting migraines) include cheese (especially aged cheese), eggs, milk (especially low-fat milk), wheat, sourdough bread, soybeans, soy sauce, tofu, corn, yeast, and many processed foods.

Interestingly, anti-seizure medications that block glutamate are used to treat both migraine and epilepsy sufferers. Even more interesting is that **ketone bodies block glutamate and therefore help to stop migraines.**

A 2013 observational study via the Department of Neurophysiology of Vision and Neurophthalmology, found that the ketogenic diet reduced migraine frequency in a whopping 90 percent of patients.

The ketogenic diet has proven to be valuable in many areas of health and this includes the improvement of those migraines.

A Potential Role for Ketone Supplements?

Emerging evidence shows that supplementing with the ketone body beta-hydroxybutyrate (BHB) may also help curb migraines, and with the ketogenic diet gaining popularity, there is strong interest in supplements containing concentrated amounts of ketones that could provide therapeutic benefits.

Chapter 11. Keto and Migraines

In 2017, at the 18th Congress of the International Headache Society, Swiss researchers presented evidence that exogenous ketone supplementation in the form of racemic ketone (BHB) salts and MCT oil were able to decrease the frequency of migraines in 5 patients studied. Although the sample size was a small group, they cut their migraine frequency in half in only 1 month. The researchers called for additional studies to help bolster the evidence that supplemental ketones can help mitigate migraines, and announced that they themselves were enrolling patients in a larger clinical trial to study the effects of supplemental BHB on migraine sufferers.

The bottom line is that both research and anecdotal evidence supports the use of the ketogenic diet and increasing interest in using ketone supplements as therapy for migraines.

Section IV

The Benefits of Ketosis on Cancer, Neurologic Diseases, Aging, and General Health and Performance

Chapter 12. Ketosis and Cancer: Exploiting the Metabolism of Cancer Cells

Cancer. Just the mention of this word sends chills down most people's spine. It's a ruthless disease that has impacted just about everyone on the planet – if not someone directly, it has likely affected a relative, loved one, or close friend. It seems like almost every month we are hearing about someone we know being diagnosed with this frightening disease.

The exact cause of cancer is not completely known, but it is multi-factorial, complex and impacted by a number of things, many of which we know, and many of which we do not know for sure. Unfortunately there is currently no sure-fire cure for cancer, although many types of cancer are treatable with surgery, radiation and/or chemotherapy and can be put into remission for years, decades, and even a lifetime. That's part of the good news. Many types of cancer are preventable and treatable, especially when discovered early, before they can metastasize and spread throughout the body. Others are incredibly aggressive, and when they impact certain organs such as the lungs, pancreas, liver, and brain, they can be incredibly difficult to fight.

What does this have to do with ketogenic therapies, the ketogenic diet and being in the state of ketosis? Well, as has been noted in the previous chapters, there is good news about keto's role in relation to cancer. **Increasingly, research is suggesting that ketones can be beneficial in the fight against cancer in a number of ways:**

1. Following a ketogenic or low-carb and no sugar diet shows potential for being preventative.

2. Certain types of cancer cells have a metabolic weakness that can be exploited by ketones and ketosis.

3. Fasting and being in the state of ketosis may have a profound effect on the immune system and stem cell production that may help the body fight certain types of cancer.

Let us be very clear – we are not saying that keto is a cure for cancer. In fact, you've probably heard or seen sensational headlines about how "cancer is addicted to sugar, so if you stop eating sugar and/or go Keto, you'll beat cancer!" There is a nugget of truth in there, but it's not nearly that simple. The promising news is that ketosis and ketogenic dieting does have a number of potential positive effects that may help you and your loved ones avoid a cancer diagnosis, or may help them in their fight cancer if they've been diagnosed with it. How is this possible? Let's dig into the science and the facts of the three areas of potential benefit mentioned above.

Ketosis and Cancer Prevention

As noted previously, cancer is a complex disease with multiple causes and factors that affect it. So what should you do if you want to do whatever you can to prevent yourself from getting cancer? Well, if we look at some of the major factors associated with cancer, a few things bubble to the surface.

Obesity. One of the most obvious links is found between cancer and obesity. Although many of the studies that link cancer and obesity are observational, and do not pinpoint specific risks, in general there is consistent evidence that higher body fat levels are associated with increased risk of many types of cancers including endometrial, esophageal, gastric, liver, kidney, pancreatic, and colorectal, among others. In fact, in many of these cancers, obesity doubled the risk of cancer.

The reasons for the link between obesity and cancer are complex, but hypotheses include the following:
(1) Hormones – fat cells produce excess estrogen, and higher levels of estrogen have been linked to increased risk of breast, endometrial, ovarian, and other cancers. In addition, obese people tend to have elevated levels of insulin and insulin-like growth factor (IGF-1). These hormones are also linked to higher incidence of several types of cancer, such as colon, endometrial, kidney, and

prostate cancers. As we discussed earlier in the book, insulin is a pro-inflammatory hormone, and it stimulates cell growth and signals fat storage. So insulin is a key player in cancer risk.

(2) Inflammation – obesity and chronic low-level inflammation go hand-in-hand, and as we discussed earlier, inflammation can damage DNA. This DNA damage as been linked to higher incidence of cancer. In addition, obese people often have other inflammatory disorders that can add to the inflammatory burden and increase the risk of certain types of cancers.

Type 2 diabetes (T2D). Closely tied to obesity (obesity and T2D are linked), and building on the damage caused by hyperinsulinemia (excess insulin levels), T2D is another risk factor. A 2018 meta-analysis of over 20 million individuals clearly showed the proven increased risk for cancer, and that the risk is slightly higher for women than men with T2D, although the significance does vary by cancer type and location. But the bottom line is, if you want to lower your risk of getting cancer, T2D is a condition to prevent and avoid. As noted above, the mechanism of incidence is linked to obesity, excess hormone levels such as insulin and IGF-1, and chronic low-level inflammation.

Of course, that's where keto comes in for obesity and diabetes. We know that low carb and ketogenic diets have been recommended for years, to help reduce body mass index (BMI), body fat levels, reverse obesity and even reverse diabetes. In 2015, a panel of experts from more than 8 countries did a critical review of the medical literature and recommended carbohydrate-restricted diets as first line therapy for diabetes and obesity. In addition, a recent clinical trial showed that nearly 60% of type 2 diabetes patients put on a ketogenic diet were able to eliminate or greatly reduce their need for medication, and effectively reversed their diabetes.

So the takeaway here is, reduce your BMI and body fat levels and if you are pre-diabetic or diabetic, start reducing your carb intake to reverse this process, stabilize your blood sugar, and lower the levels of insulin and other hormones that have been linked to increased risks of cancer.

Exploiting a Metabolic Weakness in Cancer Cells: Glucose vs Ketones

As mentioned above, you may have seen or heard sensational headlines claiming that cancer cells love sugar, and you can cure cancer by eliminating sugar from your diet. Well, curing cancer is not quite that simple, but this sensationalism does have some very sound basis in fact. So let's dig into this a bit.

Cancer cells DO love glucose.
Certain types of cancer cells (not all, however) require and use huge amounts of glucose (using a process called glycolysis described by Dr. Otto Warburg in the 1920s) in order to maintain cell respiration, generate energy, and to proliferate and spread. In fact, this abnormally high usage of glucose is key to one of the medical imaging studies used to identify cancerous regions in the body: the FDG-PET scan. That stands for flouro-deoxyglucose positron emission tomography (FDG-PET). It's the "flouro-deoxyglucose" part that is important here. What it means is, this imaging technique looks for concentrations of high glucose compared to normal glucose levels, and highlights them. Those areas light up like crazy, and that typically means there are cancerous cells accompanying those abnormally high concentrations of glucose.

Another aspect of this is that many cancer cells also have a mutation wherein they can ONLY use glucose for fuel. Your normal, healthy cells can switch to ketones as a fuel, which is what happens when you go on a ketogenic diet or use ketone supplements. But many types of cancer cells cannot do this and thus, glucose is the only fuel they can use. This metabolic weakness is something that keto may be able to exploit.

So the fact is, many types of cancer cells are reliant on glucose as an energy source. That is why there have been hypotheses that cutting off the glucose supply will "starve" cancer. And to some degree, this is the case – increasing research on cancer and keto has shown that reducing that glucose level in the body can "starve" and weaken some cancer cells, helping to slow their growth, spread, and also making them more susceptible to traditional cancer therapies like radiation and chemotherapy. So a keto diet may not "cure" cancer, but it can be an effective tool and part of a multi-pronged approach to fighting certain types of cancer. But we also want to be very factual and not overstate the potential of it as a stand-alone cure. As of this writing there is no sure-fire cure for cancer. Yet, we are hopeful that research will continue to show how ketogenic nutrition, ketone supplementation and therapies can be of benefit in the fight against this terrible disease!

On a final note, it's important to point out that not all cancers are alike, and not all are susceptible to glucose starvation. A 2018 study of preclinical evidence on the ketogenic diet and cancer showed which cancer types are and are not potentially benefited by keto. See Figure 1 below.

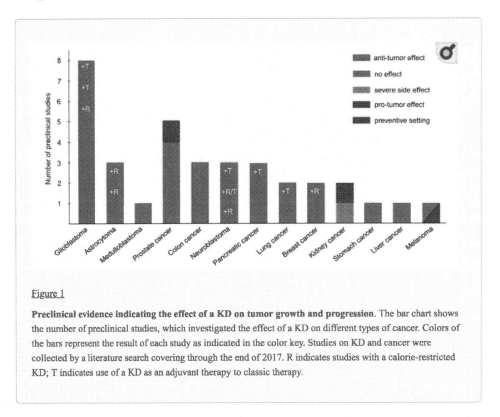

Figure 1

Preclinical evidence indicating the effect of a KD on tumor growth and progression. The bar chart shows the number of preclinical studies, which investigated the effect of a KD on different types of cancer. Colors of the bars represent the result of each study as indicated in the color key. Studies on KD and cancer were collected by a literature search covering through the end of 2017. R indicates studies with a calorie-restricted KD; T indicates use of a KD as an adjuvant therapy to classic therapy.

Figure 1. From: Weber DD, Aminazdeh-Gohari S, Kofler B. Ketogenic diet in cancer therapy. *Aging* 2018; 10(2):164-165.

Ketosis and Fasting Boost Immune Function and Gene Expression

The third aspect of ketosis and ketogenic therapies in the fight against cancer has to do with fasting, immune function and related aspects of the state of ketosis. Yale researchers a few years ago were investigating the effects of fasting that cause the body to raise its levels of blood ketones. They went on to show that the ketone beta-hydroxybutyrate (BHB) inhibits the NRLP3 inflammasome and related inflammatory diseases. So the effect of ketones on the body as a result of fasting is well noted in the scientific and medical literature. But the benefits of fasting go beyond just that.

Other research has shown that fasting reboots the immune system and protects healthy cells, which could be very useful for cancer patients who are undergoing chemotherapy. In fact some cancer centers are even suggesting that fasting prior to undergoing chemotherapy may be useful. Animal studies showed that fasting made cancer cells more susceptible to targeted radiation and chemotherapy. However, there are yet to be well-documented clinical trials in humans to verify these effects beyond the animal models.

In addition, fasting has been shown to cause the body to decrease levels of IGF-1 and PKA, and promote the regeneration of stem cells, increasing white blood cells, and reversing immunosuppression caused by chemotherapy. Again, these studies were also done in mice, but were done in multiple different cancer models, which provided more confidence that such research may be applicable to humans as well.

So in summary, ketogenic therapies are potentially effective in the prevention and treatment of cancer – but clinical studies on humans need to be done to prove the science and to provide evidence that will allow medical centers to implement it. However, they do show more promise for some types of cancer than others, so it's not a blanket that may impact all cancers.

Chapter 13. Neurologic and Cognitive Benefits of Ketones

As we've discussed earlier in the book, one of the biggest beneficial qualities of ketones is that they are a very potent energy source, providing about 38% more energy than glucose. That's why many people who are fueling themselves on ketones, whether from the ketogenic diet, intermittent fasting, exercise and/or from supplemental exogenous ketones, report having an abundance of energy. It's also the reason why so many athletes and fitness professionals, and health minded people are turning to a ketogenic lifestyle to achieve better performance. You'll soon be one of them!

That increased energy is also one of the keys to another aspect of ketones: **neurologic and cognitive benefits.** Studies have shown that the brain prefers ketones over glucose, and in fact, *ketones improve brain energy metabolism.* They also benefit brain cell mitochondria, the powerhouses of the cells. As a result, there are numerous neurologic conditions that are showing benefit from the ketogenic diet and ketogenic therapies.

In this chapter, we're going to delve into some of these, including epilepsy, depression and mood disorders, autism spectrum disorders, neuromuscular conditions such as Parkinson's and ALS, and more.

In general, ketogenic diet and lifestyle practitioners report that they feel more alert, aware, focused, and have better mental clarity when they are in ketosis. That alone makes this diet, lifestyle, and/or supplementation worth trying. From personal experience, we can attest to our own cognitive improvement from being in a ketosis-fueled heightened state of consciousness. Wouldn't you love to experience this too? It's such a great reminder that the ketogenic diet is not just a weight-loss diet. It has profound effects on daily quality of life!

That said, the therapeutic potential of ketones is massive, and we wanted to touch on some of the more common disorders that ketones have been reported to – and in many cases are being scientifically proven to – help.

Epilepsy

The ketogenic diet and epilepsy have a longstanding historical relationship, because back before the advent of anti-epilepsy drugs, the ketogenic diet was THE medical treatment for epilepsy. All the way back in the 1920s, physicians and hospitals used the ketogenic diet to treat pediatric patients who had epilepsy, and it was highly effective. When the brain is fueling on ketones, seizure activity is either stopped or greatly reduced. However, with the increasing usage of sugar, processed flour and other starches in the Western diet, keeping kids with epilepsy on a ketogenic diet was difficult. When anti-seizure drugs were developed, there was a quick movement to this easier method – why deal with the complexity of keeping a child on a strict diet when you can just give them a pill? Unfortunately, the ketogenic diet was almost completely abandoned, and became an outdated scientific footnote and little-known therapy in only a few decades.

But enter Hollywood director James Abrahams in the 1990s (you may know him from movies such as *Airplane!* and the *Naked Gun* series). His son Charlie was diagnosed with severe and almost certainly life-threatening epilepsy, having hundreds of seizures a day. Drugs were of little help. Desperate to help his son, James did some painstaking research and found out about this old, forgotten ketogenic diet, and decided to take Charlie to Johns Hopkins Medical Center, which was familiar with the diet. To make a long story short, the diet worked miraculously. Charlie's seizures stopped almost immediately, and eventually he was considered cured of his epilepsy. Charlie's amazing story and success with the diet led the family to create The Charlie Foundation for Ketogenic Therapies (www.charliefoundation.org) and even led James Abrahams to release a movie in 1994 about the ketogenic diet that starred Meryl Streep. You can watch it here: https://www.youtube.com/watch?v=2_8D1hH7mzo

In the past couple of decades, increasing incidence of drug-resistant seizures has led to a resurgent interest in the ketogenic diet as a therapeutic solution, and many leading medical centers and hospitals in the U.S. and around the world are offering ketogenic diet guidance as well as other ketogenic therapies. So you can rest assured that your desire to try the ketogenic diet is backed by the medical community.

Another interesting historical story about ketones and seizures has to do with the creation of supplemental ketones. The department of defense was aware of the anti-seizure qualities of ketones and funded researchers to come up with a ketone supplement that would mitigate the risk of seizure activity in Navy seals who were scuba diving using high-oxygen rebreathers (a stealth mode of diving that does not produce location giveaway bubbles). When oxygen is under pressure, which happens at depth underwater, it can become toxic to the brain and result in seizures that can happen without warning, and can be fatal for obvious reasons if one is 100 feet underwater and has a seizure.

The researchers did develop a ketone supplement and it led to some unexpected results – the volunteers who used it reported feeling higher levels of energy, focus, and mental clarity and alertness. This was the beginning of the development of exogenous ketone supplements, which are now only recently available to the general public.

For more information about how ketones can help epilepsy and seizure disorders, google "ketogenic diet and epilepsy" or "ketones and epilepsy" and you'll be inundated with scientific articles and websites. One of the most comprehensive web sites that explains how keto can treat epilepsy is that of the Charlie Foundation: https://charliefoundation.org/keto-for-epilepsy/

Alzheimer's and Dementia

An extremely exciting and promising area of ketogenic benefit is the ability for ketones to help Alzheimer's and dementia patients. To be clear, there is no cure for these diseases, but there is increasing clinical research and anecdotal evidence showing that putting these patients on a high-fat, low-carb ketogenic diet, MCT oil supplements, and/or supplemental exogenous ketones, can result in improvement of their cognitive capabilities and cognitive assessment scores.

A 2018 pilot study using the ketogenic diet and MCT (medium chain triglycerides) supplements on a group of patients with mild Alzheimer's disease showed that the cognitive test results improved significantly in 9 out of 10 participants, and so the researchers are looking into larger studies to help validate the results. Interestingly, the patients who returned to a non-ketogenic diet saw their cognitive improvement disappear as well.

Because Alzheimer's is considered by many as "type 3 diabetes" and is believed to be impacted by insulin resistance, elevated glucose levels, and hyperinsulinemia, keto makes a lot of sense for these patients. We know that the ketogenic diet can positively improve and even reverse diabetes, and so it goes to follow that keto would benefit these patients by mitigating those risk factors. In addition, as discussed in previous chapters, ketone bodies improve brain energy metabolism, and thus may help to improve cognition in patients with Alzheimer's and dementia. Unfortunately, the ketogenic diet and other ketogenic therapies are not a cure, but in the opinion of the authors, they should be strongly considered as part of the treatment protocol for Alzheimer's and dementia patients. In addition, we believe that individuals who hope to stave off the development of these diseases would be wise to consider the ketogenic lifestyle for prevention, and we hope to see research conducted that would validate these preventative hypotheses. Any diet that can help improve cognitive ability and assessment scores and improve the way your brain generates and uses energy, seems like a good idea, don't you think?

Mood and Brain Disorders (Depression, Anxiety, Bipolar and Schizophrenia)

Because of the ketogenic diet's usefulness in treating epilepsy, a number of other brain disorders have been hypothesized to potentially benefit from keto. Among them are mood disorders such as depression and anxiety, and brain disorders such as bipolar and schizophrenia. The reason these disorders are hypothesized to potentially benefit from ketogenic treatments is primarily due to the impact of ketones on improving brain energy metabolism, as mentioned previously. There are many anecdotal reports of people who felt their depression improved or completely disappeared once they started a ketogenic diet or began supplementing with beta-hydroxybutyrate, spurring hypotheses that the ketogenic diet and/or increased levels of ketones fueling the brain, may hold anti-depressant properties.

Unfortunately at this time, no randomized clinical trials have been completed to date on humans, but there are some in the investigative stages. Animal studies have proven to be very positive, however. Anxiety has been studied in rat models with a lot of promise being shown in ketone supplementation reducing anxiety and related stress models in Sprague-Dawley rats. Similar studies on the ketogenic diet have shown improvement in bipolar disorders and schizophrenia in rats, and some small case studies in humans have caused increased interest in larger clinical trials.

That said, the increasing number of people using the ketogenic diet should make it easier to do clinical trials to determine a connection, if one exists, and to provide support for the hypotheses around keto being an anti-depressant of sorts.

Autism Spectrum Disorders

Autism spectrum disorders are typically neurodevelopmental disorders with hallmarks of impaired social communication capabilities, coupled with restricted or repetitive behaviors. Many patients with these disorders have specific interests or foci of behavior. They often also have adverse behaviors that include attention deficits, anxiety, inability to focus, and even self-inflicted injury or injury toward others when agitated. There is a very wide range of ability to function with some patients needing intensive ongoing care and others capable of normal lifestyle with minor intervention or limitations.

Behavioral therapies are typically intensive and pharmaceutical therapies often have significant side effects. It's no wonder that there has been a desire to look into the cause and treatment of these disorders as the incidence continues to increase worldwide.

As we've discussed in this chapter already, many neurological disorders respond positively to carbohydrate restriction (especially sugar restriction) and ketogenic nutrition. In autism spectrum disorders specifically, there have been numerous animal studies as well as human case reports and studies showing the potential benefit of the ketogenic diet. The science underlying most of this is the role ketones play in optimizing the mitochondria of brain cells.

A recent clinical trial in 15 children in Honolulu that combined a ketogenic diet with MCT oil supplementation showed significant improvement in their core autism features, especially social affective components (fear, anxiety, and imitation). The researchers have called for broader studies to help better understand how ketogenic nutrition and therapies can play a role in treatment for patients with autism spectrum disorders.

To be clear, keto is not a cure for autism, but as with Alzheimer's and dementia, it can improve cognitive and behavioral function, and we would recommend that caregivers of autistic patients consider investigating the use of a ketogenic diet and/or ketogenic therapies to improve their patients' symptoms.

One caveat is that autistic individuals often don't tolerate changes to their routine and habits, so introducing a new diet and getting adherence to that diet may be challenging. It may be easier to introduce exogenous ketone supplementation as a potential first step, to assess any changes or benefits before attempting to make significant dietary changes.

Parkinson's, ALS, and Other Neuromotor Disorders

Ever since scientists showed that epilepsy could be treated and even cured with a ketogenic diet, researchers have looked at other brain-oriented conditions that could potentially be benefitted by the ketogenic diet. Among them are Parkinson's disease, ALS, and other neuromotor and neuromuscular disorders.

Keto and Parkinson's Disease

Parkinson's disease is a result of the deterioration of the cells in the brain that produce dopamine, and the cause of it is unknown. Patients with the disease often suffer from mild to severe tremors, rigidity of muscles, and slow movement. As the disease progresses, they can experience difficulty speaking, moving, and walking, as well as emotional issues, depression, and even dementia. The drugs that treat Parkinson's typically have a lot of side effects and can lose their effectiveness over time. So the potential for diet to play a role in improving the quality of life in Parkinson's patients is currently being investigated.

Back in 2000, an *in vitro* study showed that the ketone body beta-hydroxybutyrate protected neurons in models of Alzheimer's and Parkinson's disease:

> *"The ability of ketone bodies to protect neurons in culture suggests that defects in mitochondrial energy generation contribute to the pathophysiology of both brain diseases. These findings further suggest that ketone bodies may play a therapeutic role in these most common forms of human neurodegeneration."*

In addition, other models of these brain diseases have shown potential promise, including case reports of patients who benefitted and saw a reduction in symptom severity when adhering to a ketogenic diet.

One published clinical study tested the effects of the ketogenic diet on symptoms of Parkinson's disease. In this non-control group study of 7 patients (5 of whom adhered to the diet), the Parkinson's disease patients had a mean of 43% reduction in Unified Parkinson's Disease Rating Scale scores after 28 days on the ketogenic diet. All participating patients reported moderate to very good improvement in symptoms. However, the limited structure of the study and small patient group suggests larger scale studies are needed.

Keto and ALS

Amyotrophic lateral sclerosis (ALS, also previously called Lou Gehrig's disease) is a rapidly progressive degenerative disease impacting the motor neurons of the cortex and anterior horn of the spinal cord. As a result, motor activity and strength deteriorate, leaving the patient progressively weaker and weaker, even though their cognitive function remains intact.

Although there is very little scientific research on keto and ALS, there remains a hypothesis that there could be potential benefit for many of the same reasons ketones may be beneficial in other neurologic diseases: the improvement of brain energy metabolism as well as neuro-protection, and the impact on mitochrondrial functioning. Unfortunately, it has been suggested that in most anecdotal cases, diseases like ALS have been too far into their progression for ketones to have any profound impact, and it's been suggested that studies need to be done on patients with early-onset ALS to determine if there are benefits to be seen.

Stroke and Traumatic Brain Injury

It has also been hypothesized that keto could help in certain aspects of brain function deficits caused by ischemia, stroke, and traumatic brain injury. There have been numerous studies of stroke and brain injury models where infusing with exogenous beta-hydroxybutyrate BEFORE the stroke or brain injury resulted in neuro-protection and lessening of severity of the injury. Likewise, some brain injuries lead to seizure activity and epileptic events. Keto has been shown to effectively decrease or prevent epileptic and certain other types of seizure activity, although studies on this after brain injury has occurred have been mixed.

Currently to our knowledge there have been no human clinical trials to date exploring whether the ketogenic diet or exogenous ketones supplied *after* an injury or stroke event would help repair other brain damage or injury, although animal studies suggest this is a possibility, and some studies have shown benefit to giving a post-injury ketogenic diet. The mechanism for this is not completely understood, but is thought to be most likely due to the ability of ketones to cross the blood-brain barrier and improve brain energy metabolism. In addition, many types of brain injury result in an impaired ability for brain cells to use glucose effectively as energy, and so ketones may bypass this impairment and provide much needed energy to brain cell mitochondria. Brain injury also often results in oxidative stress, which ketones have been shown to alleviate and repair. And recently, research has shown that ketones help to stabilize brain networks and fill the energy gap between what the brain needs and what energy is being supplied.

Chapter 13. Neurologic and Cognitive Benefits of Ketones

As in other brain and neurologic conditions, just the fact that ketones can improve brain energy metabolism and reduce oxidative stress is enough to warrant some to suggest trying exogenous ketones or ketogenic diets in an attempt to alleviate symptoms of brain injuries and stroke. The conventional wisdom being that it can't hurt, so why not try it? That said, at this time there is little in terms of evidence-based clinical research that would prove any benefit, so any expectations of keto and a cure or significant treatment for stroke and TBI should be tempered until more research is done.

Finally, although patient studies are currently not available, many of these traumatic brain injury and depressive mood disorder benefits are believed to be helpful for PTSD patients who often have suffered both physical and psychological trauma. Anecdotal reports have been positive, but as of this writing, clinical studies have not been performed.

Summary

Scientific and clinical research is increasingly showing that ketones (especially BHB) and the ketogenic diet have great potential to impact brain, neurologic and mood disorders. Although some benefits, like seizure reduction in epilepsy, are clearly proven, other areas sorely need more clinical research – on humans, not rodents or cell cultures – and more structured dose-dependent studies to effectively determine whether ketogenic diets and/or supplements can have a profound and meaningful therapeutic effect. However, we the authors feel there is enough clinical, hypothetical and anecdotal evidence to encourage the use of the ketogenic therapies outlined in *The Ketogenic Key*. The bottom line is, this is new, exciting, and very promising!

Chapter 14. Ketones and Aging: Improving Longevity, Lifespan, and Healthspan

What's the secret to improving longevity, aging, and healthspan? And can ketosis help?

You may be thinking that longevity is essentially winning the genetic lottery. Our genes do have a role in our life span, however, it is our environment (namely our choices) that we are placed in that plays a powerful and much bigger role than the genes we were born with.

For many people, if asked how long they want to live, their answer is "not too long." The reason for this answer is that generally, people who live a long life are not healthy toward the end of their life, and may be ill and suffer for many years before they die.

The key is to not only extend our *lifespan,* but our *healthspan* as well. Supporting the biological mechanisms to longevity with ketosis, for example, may well do that by removing metabolic blocks.

How Ketosis Can Optimize Longevity

The premise of using ketosis for longevity is that when carbohydrate intake is drastically lowered, or stopped entirely, the body must find a new primary source of energy.

Research shows that calorie restriction, without malnutrition (in mice) has been shown to increase lifespan and healthspan and this is a result of a shift away from glucose dependent diets towards a fat-adapted metabolism. The mice on higher fat diets had longer lives, lower midlife mortality rates, and performed better on tests pertaining to certain cognitive functioning.

One theory that purports to extend longevity and health is by taking care of our mitochondria. As we outline in the Hallmarks of

Chapter 14. Ketones and Aging

Aging [below], our mitochondria produce energy, and being in ketosis has a powerful impact upon these ubiquitous and crucial tiny cellular engines. Damage to our mitochondria has a broad impact upon the cellular systems within the body and hasten the demise of the organism.

However, simply eating a low-carb diet packed with whole foods and one that exemplifies the qualities of the ketogenic diet, for example, provides us with many protective benefits from common and age-related conditions associated with poor diet, such as heart disease, diabetes, and obesity.

Hallmarks of Aging

So what is aging? The last few decades have witnessed tremendous developments in the understanding of the aging process. Aging can be broadly described as the progressive, time-dependent deterioration of cellular function caused by the accumulation of cellular damage.

There are many theories but essentially despite the theory, aging leaves its imprint in a generally typical effect on humans.

In fact, the Hallmarks of Aging is the name of a 2013 paper published in the journal *Cell* and it describes the nine broad categories of cellular and molecular damage that are generally accepted to be the causes of aging. In other words, it describes essentially the process of human degradation.

It is important to note that the hallmarks don't exist in isolation – in other words, they influence each other. So, what are they? Primary hallmarks of aging are thought to be the triggers of age-related decline and their effects, which accumulate with time and are negative.

Here is a List of the Commonly Recognized Hallmarks of Aging:

1. Genomic Instability.

Each cell contains all of the instructions it needs to create a healthy cell and its function. For this reason, you wouldn't want your genome to be damaged, as this would change the way the cell performs and it would create terrible consequences. This is why your genome is stored away in the cell's nucleus safe from harm.

Unfortunately, damage can occur such as accumulated mutations from internal or external factors such as excess UV light or viral infections or even internal factors as each time your cell divides, they make a copy of themselves (the cell) all the way down to the genome and copies are never like the original and change with each replication in some small way.

Protecting the genome is crucial and why we have built-in protective repair mechanisms. But despite these in-place protections, mutations and more can impact the integrity of the original cell's replication and as we grow older, we accumulate more damage to the DNA. This can interfere with stem cell activity, tissue repair and even result in mutations such as cancer.

It doesn't stop there. Mitochondria, the tiny powerhouses that make energy without which we would not be alive, have their own genome and are exponentially prone to damage, as they are part of the energy creation of a cell and exposed to oxidative stress. Additionally, the mitochondria have a lousy DNA repair mechanism compared to that of the DNA in the cell nucleus, and that's why it is crucial to keep mitochondria healthy.

Damage to the mitochondria is very serious and is referred to as Mitochondrial Dysfunction that leads not only to faster aging, *but poor health outcomes such as illness and disease.*

2. Telomeres

You may have heard of telomeres before, as they are often compared to the plastic aglet tips on the ends of a shoelace. The reason for these protective "caps" of repeated segments of DNA is to serve as chromosomal safeguards from damage and deterioration or even fusing with other chromosomes.

The problem is, every time a cell divides, the telomere length shortens with each division until eventually there is virtually no length (called the "Hayflick Limit"). The cell no longer can replicate (becomes senescent) leading to even more cellular dysfunction within the body in most cases.

Cellular senescence is a stress response triggered by many factors associated with aging such as genomic instability and telomere attrition, which are, again, primary aging hallmarks themselves.

In humans, shorter telomeres represent a health risk, even if young.

3. Epigenetics

Along with our genome, we also have an epigenome – a collection of chemical compounds that act as switches. If the switch is on, the gene will be expressed, which means the protein that the gene encodes for will be expressed. However, if the gene is "silent," that gene will not be expressed, because the protein for that gene was not produced.

You can look at the epigenome as the software and the gene as the hardware. This is where the aforementioned environment is crucial. Our choices such as the food we eat, the toxins we are exposed to, chronic stress or lack of sleep, for example, determine which genes are silenced and which genes are switched on. Our genome is essentially stable. However, our epigenome is not, and these environmentally caused changes in the epigenome can accumulate over a lifetime, weakening the immune system, potentially causing cancer, and contributing to low-grade inflammation. More generally, they negatively affect the proper functioning of your cells.

4. Loss of Proteostasis

The wide-scale loss of protein homeostasis (proteostasis), the way protein molecules serve many key roles in the body, is thought to be one of the primary hallmarks of aging. The correct functioning of proteins, despite their size, is a key player in how well we age.

Protein aggregation and mis-folding are associated with many age-related disorders, and increased protein oxidation. To avoid this problem, cells have mechanisms that promote correct protein folding and other mechanisms that break down mis-folded proteins and recycle their components.

Research has shown that our ability to maintain proteostasis diminishes with age, again, leading to an accumulation of broken proteins that can contribute to the development of many age-related diseases such as Alzheimer's disease, Parkinson's disease, and cataracts.

5. Mitochondrial Dysfunction

Mitochondria are microscopic organelles that operate in large numbers within your cells. Their job is to produce a molecule called ATP (adenosine triphosphate), which is then used to power all types of cellular functions.

Mitochondria can be damaged in more than one way. For example, chronic stresses, chronic sleep loss, unhealthy food choices, and much more. Dysfunctional mitochondria produce less ATP, which means less energy supplied to the cell. Mitochondrial dysfunction is considered a hallmark of aging that does accelerate aging. Additionally, a natural reduction in the number of mitochondria occurs as we age, and that contributes to aging.

6. Cellular Senescence

Cellular senescence means that the cell is no longer able to divide. This also means it is not functioning but still active in its ability to help with wound healing, which serves a useful purpose. However, as with most hallmarks of aging, it is the accumulation that is the catalyst and such is the case for senescent cells; it is the accumulation of them that is unhealthy for you. As we noted earlier, the shortening of telomeres promotes the cell's demise and other factors such as damage to the chromosome.

We know that if a cell's DNA is damaged, it can malfunction and turn cancerous, and senescence puts a halt to cell replication and creates damaged cells. Once a cell becomes senescent, it is usually destroyed by the immune system.

Senescent cells can be beneficial, such as in wound healing, yet the accumulation of them emits a cascade of inflammatory-type signals or chemicals that spread to healthy cells, causing distress, systemic inflammation and deterioration, which is why researchers believe that removal of senescent cells may radically change medicine.

The problem is that the mechanism for senescent cells falters with age, so they don't get cleared as efficiently as they did when the body is younger. Additionally, senescent cells need to be replaced, but are not due to their senescence, and this too contributes to the aging process.

In mouse studies, cellular senescence has been implicated in a vast array of age-related diseases including arthritis and cancer. Scientists think this also might be true for humans.

7. Deregulated Nutrient Sensing

In order for our bodies to carry on the basics of living, cells need to use key nutrients. Cells are highly evolved to "sense" when nutrients are around. Signals tell the cell to grow and utilize these nutrients.

Some of these nutrient signals work to promote growth and metabolism acceleration of cells in the body during the times that nutrients such as glucose are abundant, which promotes aging. Other signals do just the opposite.

One example of the accelerator signal is the insulin pathway, which tells the cells there is an abundance of glucose in your blood. Research has shown that specific pathways such as insulin-like growth factors have been reduced and theorized this may be an adaptive response to accumulated cellular damage.

It may be that when we are in ketosis, and glucose is not abundant, that our cells sense that these nutrients are not abundance, and thus slow down the aging mechanisms. It has been shown that reducing nutrients via intermittent fasting, calorie restriction and other means, resulted in longevity in studies on certain types of yeasts and mice. We need additional studies to show this happens in humans, but the hypothesis is there.

8. Stem Cell Exhaustion

Stem cells are basically what of all of your cells originate from. Normally, each cell in your body has a role; it can be a heart cell, a muscle cell, a brain cell and so on. But stem cells are basically blank and haven't been coded to take up any role yet.

One example of aging shows up as our body's ability to replace damaged tissues slows down as time goes on. This can affect every tissue in our body from our skin to our organs, and even our immune system, which is called immunosenescence – the weakening of the immune system as we age. The reason this happens is that with age, the body slowly runs out of stem cells. Additionally, chronic inflammation (that is common with aging) can impair and inhibit the cells' ability to divide. Also, interference from other aging hallmarks is what makes stem cell exhaustion an important hallmark on its own.

9. Altered Cellular Communication

We might be inclined to think that each aging hallmark only affects a specific system such as the mitochondria or stem cells. Unfortunately, aging affects all systems, not just individual cells or systems, and it affects the way the different components interact with each other.

In order for your body to function, the cells and organs need to communicate. There are many ways aging can interfere with cellular communication in a broad way within the body.

A prominent feature of the aging process within altered cellular communication is inflammation, or what is aptly referred to as *inflamm-aging.* This is a chronic and systemic low-grade inflammatory process. Inflammation is due to a number of factors that increase as you age such as the accumulation of damaged tissues presenting itself as osteoarthritis, for example.

As an acute short-lived immune response reaction, inflammation is a healthy reaction. Chronic inflammation, however, has been shown to contribute to age-related diseases including type 2 diabetes, atherosclerosis and even cancer. This is because inflammation interferes with the normal activity of your immune system – not only impairing one's ability to deal with bacteria and viruses, but also by blocking out its ability to clear out cancer cells.

Aged tissue can effect and damage surrounding healthy cells in a type of cascade reaction, similar to senescent cells. By protecting and delaying inflammation in specific tissues, you are also protecting healthy surrounding tissues.

Ketosis to the Rescue? Mitigation of Aging Hallmarks

This is where ketosis comes into the equation. An increasing number of studies are showing that ketone bodies help mimic and support anti-aging processes within the body. As we mentioned earlier in the book, one of the things that ketosis does, is trick your body into thinking it is starving. So ketone bodies have been shown to mimic the anti-aging properties of calorie-restriction. In addition, by reducing inflammation (the ketone body BHB has been shown to inhibit NLRP3 inflammasome-mediated inflammation), being in ketosis reduces some of the factors that contribute to the hallmarks of aging. Intermittent fasting has been shown to boost the immune system and even help the body generate stem cells. So the components of the Ketogenic Key program essentially help your body fight the processes of aging!

Chapter 15. Energy and Human Performance Benefits

As we've been pointing out already, there is so much more to the being in ketosis than just weight and fat loss. In addition to the many benefits we've already discussed, we want to address some of the benefits keto can have on your general health and well being. For example, how ketones provide a markedly increased level of energy. Then we'll discuss the impact it can have on sports, activities, and athletic performance, especially endurance sports and activities like cycling, running, rowing and more!

Ketones and Energy Levels

When discussing ketosis, ketone supplements, and the ketogenic diet, the topic of increased energy often comes up. And although this sounds a little vague, it actually has a very logical scientific reason for why people report having considerably more energy when they achieve ketosis from following a ketogenic diet or consuming therapeutic ketone supplements. And the reason for that is, ketones generate more energy than glucose or protein. In fact, ketones produce over a third more energy per gram. So the simple fact is, ketones are a more potent fuel for your body and brain.

Remember when you had science class and you studied the cells of the body? Let's have a real simple refresher. Your cells all contain a power plant in them, called the mitochondria. These cellular powerhouses are responsible for generating the energy (adenosine triphosphate, or ATP) that keeps us going. Well, ketones actually produce 38% more ATP than glucose. So it has a profound impact in terms of our energy levels when we are fueling our body and brains with ketones instead of sugar or glucose. It's like burning rocket fuel instead of kindling!

One of the reasons that the ketogenic diet optimizes your energy levels is that the ketogenic diet is high in fat. So you are eating more fats, and fat is more calorically dense than carbs and protein. A gram of fat has 9 calories while a gram of carbohydrate or protein has only 4 calories. So when you go keto, not only are you fueling your body with ketones, which pack an energetic punch, you're also consuming more calorically dense food in the fats that make up the majority of the ketogenic diet! This one-two punch means your body and brain have plenty of energy to keep going all day, without the mid-day crash and brain fog that most people experience.

Part of the reason for this steady state of energy is that ketones and fats don't cause a spike in blood sugar, so they help keep blood glucose stable. This means more steady energy levels as well as less insulin circulating in the bloodstream, which also helps keep energy levels stable and silent inflammation low. The bottom line is that keto optimizes and maximizes your body's creation and use of energy!

This is why we recommend keto so strongly – who doesn't need more energy? Whether you're a student who needs to study long hours and attend classes, a worker who has a 9-5 schedule or shift work, a business executive who needs to be sharp and on point all day, a stay at home parent juggling kids and house work, or whatever the case, ketosis is for YOU. Most people who are in ketosis report a sense of wonderment when they can simply go all day and not burn out, crash, or hit that mid-day slump that so many people experience every day.

Ketones and Sports/Athletic Performance

As you can imagine, the benefits of increased energy noted in the previous section also apply to sports, physical activities, and athletic pursuits. More and more coaches, trainers, and athletes are moving to high-fat ketogenic diets because they understand the energy benefit that running on ketones and fat can mean to an athlete. In addition, more and more sports research is showing that many athletes perform better and more consistently when they become fat-adapted (they have shifted their body into using fat for fuel instead of glucose and sugar).

In addition, exogenous ketones (ketone supplements) have been known as a great tool for high-performance endurance athletes for a while now. In fact, in the last couple of Tour de France races, multiple teams were experimenting with exogenous ketones. In 2018, rumors were circulating (and later confirmed) that Team Sky, the winning team, supplemented with ketones (they are perfectly legal as a natural substance, but very few people understood their potential to help endurance athletes recover). But, success breeds imitation, and by 2019, a large number of the Tour teams were using exogenous ketones. These elite athletes and their trainers now know the power, benefit, and advantage of having ketones and fat fueling them during this grueling race.

In addition to reports like these, some interesting clinical sports performance research has been coming out as well. A study of elite rowers showed that those who fueled themselves with ketone supplements saw a 2% improvement in performance times. Now, that may not sound like a lot, but in athletic competitions where mere seconds or tenths of seconds mean the difference between winning, placing, and not even being part of the top 10, a 2% improvement can catapult you into the winner's circle!

In the realm of ultra-endurance racing, where competitors run for 24 hours straight, keto and fat adaption have become increasingly common as these athletes have realized how much more energy they have by using fat for fuel rather than carbs, which burn much more quickly and need constant replenishing.

An area of sports medicine in which ketones are showing great promise is neuroprotection against traumatic brain injuries (i.e., concussions) as well as CTE, which is a deterioration of the brain caused by repeated head trauma from contact sports like football. Studies are showing that the ketogenic diet not only helps protect the brain from damage, but also helps heal damage after it happens. Whether this is due to the anti-inflammatory effects of ketone bodies (discussed in an earlier chapter) or some other mechanism is not quite yet clear, but the emerging research is promising and the hope is that it leads to potential preventative and treatment options in the future, through diet and supplementation.

The bottom line is that ketones have a lot of potential in athletics and sports performance. After all, what athlete wouldn't benefit from having more energy and mental clarity and focus? Anecdotally, many different types of athletes, from golfers to

Chapter 15. Energy and Human Performance Benefits

basketball players to mixed martial arts (MMA) fighters, have adopted ketones, ketogenic nutrition and techniques such as fasting in order to help them perform at a higher level.

So as you can see, there are so many benefits to ketones, why would anyone NOT want to give the ketogenic diet, intermittent fasting, and/or ketone supplementation a try?

Section V: Getting Started With And Maintaining *The Ketogenic Key* Lifestyle!

Chapter 16. Getting Started With *The Ketogenic Key* Lifestyle

Say "Hello" to Keto!

Getting started on the Ketogenic Key lifestyle is simple: just dive in! We use terms like "lifestyle" rather than "diet," because the word "diet" implies a temporary way of eating, and pigeonholes the focus onto food only. As we have explained in this book, we recommend combining dietary changes, intermittent fasting, ketone supplementation, and exercise to optimally achieve and maintain a healthy Ketogenic Key lifestyle!

We believe that the Ketogenic Key lifestyle can be easy and fun to start, maintain, and sustain throughout your lifetime. We also believe that starting a new way of eating, like adopting a low-carb, ketogenic diet, is a great time to clean out your kitchen and replace all the old, unhealthy foods with new foods that will take you to ketogenic success. Clean out your pantry, refrigerator, desk, handbag, nightstand or any other area that you may have foods stored that can kick you out of ketosis. Remember, when you surround yourself with healthy foods, you are far more likely to eat healthy foods.

As you know by now, the ketogenic diet is a way of eating that is high in fat, moderate in protein and VERY low in carbohydrates. And just to reiterate, any type of ketogenic therapies, such as intermittent fasting, provide a bounty of benefits. It can be intimidating to start any new way of eating, and we get it. We've been doing this for many years and so we have the combined experience to help you avoid the mistakes we have made. Our stories are in the Introduction, in case you missed them!

Let's begin!

To recap, the Ketogenic Key lifestyle has numerous benefits, including:

Chapter 19

- Weight loss
- Stable mood & energy levels
- Blood sugar control
- Reduced cravings & appetite suppression
- Lower blood pressure
- Higher good cholesterol
- Skin improvements
- Digestive support
- Possibly even increased lifespan!

With the Ketogenic Key plan, our main goal is to get you into the metabolic state called *ketosis* in which the body burns fat and ketones for fuel. Your mission is to arrive at this state and begin to create efficient metabolic machinery that will optimize your health and weight.

How does keto differ from other low-carb eating strategies? Simple: there are different variations of a low-carb diet, and the keto diet is a special type of low carb diet with added nuances. The number of carbohydrates you can eat and still achieve ketosis will vary depending on things such as your insulin tolerance, how dependent or sensitive your body is upon carbohydrates, and your activity level, but on average, here are the common numbers of carbs allowed in well-formulated low carb diets:

- **Keto diet**: Less than 25g *net carbs* per day
- **Low carb diet**: 50g – 75g net carbs per day
- **Moderate low carb diet**: 75g – 100g net carbs per day

As you can see, the ketogenic diet requires a much lower level of carbohydrate consumption that what are typically considered "low carb" diets.

Some people opt to track their consumption of carbs diligently and some choose to simply focus on only eating low carb and keto-friendly foods. Initially, we have found through experience, that tracking carbs to get into ketosis is key for success.

Getting started in any endeavor means to **plan and prepare**, which equates to success. It is also important to have a long-term mindset. There is nothing that is a "quick fix" if done in a healthy way.

Step One: Detox Your Kitchen!

The very first action step is to detox your kitchen of all junk foods (you know what they are): foods that call your name while you're in the other room, and any and all unhealthy foods, period. Remember, you are a product of your environment. We all have our vulnerable times when changing to a new eating style. So surrounding yourself only with the foods from the Ketogenic Key food list will help keep you successful in achieving and maintaining ketosis. Some people are concerned about the cost of eating keto friendly foods, but in our experience, when you eat a high-fat diet, you are satiated more and actually eat less food than when you are eating a standard American diet. That said, if you have a large family or want to conserve dollars, consider buying your meats, veggies and other items in bulk and freezing them, as that can help you save money and ensures you have plenty of good keto foods around.

Step Two: Track Those Carbs!

Next, you want to begin to track your consumption of carbohydrates. In our experience, the folks who track carbs are the ones who are most successful. Why is this? Well, it's easy to overeat carbs, even when eating low-carb foods. For example, if you know that pecans are low in carbs, you may be tempted to eat a few more than the suggested serving size. This means that in the process of transitioning to or staying in ketosis, eating those extra nuts could be a make or break choice. You may find yourself surprised as to how many carbs are lurking in so many foods. This is why it is vital to read labels, and to track the carbs you are eating!

Fortunately there are many tools available that make carb tracking a snap! The app *MyFitnessPal* is an excellent tool that provides quick keto assistance on the nutritional value of most every food. Ideally, you would want to track:

- Carbohydrates
- Fat
- Fiber

- Protein
- Potassium

In fact, there is an excellent online article about how to customize MyFitnessPal for the keto diet. You can find it at:

https://www.ruled.me/carb-tracking-for-keto-diet/

Starting out, we do not recommend that you focus on tracking calories when transitioning or staying in ketosis. Eating until you are full using the Ketogenic Key foods list and keeping your carbs low, will make the transition much more sustainable long-term. For example, eating an omelet for breakfast or at anytime, will keep you satiated. If you find your weight loss progress slowing or plateauing, then it might be helpful to start calorie tracking as well. When eating high-fat foods that are dense in calories such as nuts, it is sometimes easy to over-eat them without realizing it. It is important to make sure you are creating an energy deficit (more on this later in the chapter) so that you tap into your stored body fat for energy.

Are You In Ketosis?

Once you are well into the Ketogenic Key lifestyle, ketosis will happen – just remember that everyone is different, and everyone's body keto-adapts at a different speed. It can happen within days or weeks when the ketogenic diet is followed correctly as this will raise your blood ketone levels. On a ketogenic diet, your body undergoes many biological adaptations, including a reduction in blood glucose, insulin levels and increased fat breakdown.

When this happens, your liver starts breaking down fat to produce ketones to supply energy for your body and brain. But how do you know when you've hit that sweet ketotic spot? There are definite signs! Please note that some of these may appear to be undesirable, but mostly are temporary as your body switches from glucose to ketones and has to adapt to this new fuel source. We call this becoming "keto-adapted." After all, you've been fueling your body on glucose since you were an infant, so it's expected that there will be a few weeks of time that your body needs to transition to a new – but far superior – fuel source!

Chapter 16. Getting Started With The Ketogenic Key Lifestyle

Here are common signs you are in ketosis:

1. **Appetite Suppression.** Ketones have been shown to have a mild appetite suppression effect. This means you will easily say no to unhealthy foods that called your name in the past. Hunger or cravings are history.
2. **Fat Loss.** When you severely restrict carbs, faster weight loss is a common result – note that we specifically say "fat loss", because ultimately we are trying to lose fat, not weight.
3. **Increased Focus and Energy.** Many people find being in ketosis gives them extraordinary clarity, energy and focus. This makes sense, as ketones are a preferred form of fuel for your body and brain compared to glucose. In fact, even in people who have both glucose and ketones in their system, the brain will preferentially use ketones for fuel. It's also a higher yield fuel. Ketones produce about 38% more ATP than glucose (ATP is the fuel your mitochondria use for energy!)
4. **Increased Thirst.** As insulin levels decrease while following a low-carb plan, the body starts expelling excess sodium and water. This may result in higher-than-normal thirst, either detected or undetected. Ensure you are drinking a minimum of half your body weight in water (with a pinch of sea salt). To balance electrolytes, we recommend adding 2 grams of sodium per day to your diet when following an extremely low-carb plan.
5. **Temporary Transient Fatigue.** One of the main issues when switching from a more glucose dependent diet to a low-carb diet is an initial period of short-term fatigue, low energy, and brain fog that can occur. This occurs during the keto-adaptation period due to the loss of electrolytes from this release of water. This is prevented when you have adequate sodium, potassium and magnesium. Again, this is temporary and will resolve over time.
6. **Changes in Workout Performance.** When beginning the ketogenic diet or any type of very low carb eating plan, for the first couple of weeks you may experience sub-optimal exercise performance that will bounce back once the body is accustomed to another (your new) source of fuel – fat. We discuss this more in our section about the "keto flu". However, once you are in ketosis and fully keto-adapted, it is highly likely you will experience an increase in stamina, endurance, and energy levels. This is due to the fact that ketones supply 38% more ATP than

glucose, so they are a higher yield fuel. In addition, when you are in ketosis, your body produces less lactic acid during exercise, and improves your respiratory output (you create less CO_2). All these things together may improve your metabolic efficiency and that in turn can manifest as improved athletic performance.

7. **Increase in Blood Ketones and Drop in Blood Glucose Levels** – A main indication of ketosis is an increase in the level of ketones in the blood and a reduction of blood glucose levels. This is a positive achievement since we know glucose levels are tied to insulin resistance, diabetes, fat accumulation, and low-level chronic inflammation.

8. **Increased Ketones in Breath or Urine** – Another way to measure ketones are with the fairly accurate breath analyzers that measure acetone, which exits the body through your breath when you are in ketosis. However, you have to use a formula to calculate how much breath acetone = ketone levels. Although it's fairly accurate, it does require some work to figure out how deep into ketosis you are. The other way is to measure urine ketones using readily available ketone urine strips from any pharmacy (they are sold with diabetes products). The thing about urine ketone levels is they are only measuring what your body is excreting, not what's actually circulating in your blood, so they are not a completely reliable method of measuring ketosis. What they do tell you is that there are ketones present. For some people, this is enough. For others, they want a more specific and accurate measurement. The gold standard for measurement however, is testing blood ketones.

9. **Digestive Changes.** Switching from one type of diet to another can cause digestive distress such as diarrhea or constipation, initially. If this happens, don't worry. Eventually your body will normalize once you've become keto-adapted and your body adjusts to eating more fat, and fewer carbohydrates. If you are using ketone supplements, you may find that ketone salts help relieve constipation. In fact, in some people, eating a lot of fat "cleans their pipes" to put it politely. Eventually your body will adapt and normalize, just give it time.

10. **Better Sleep.** Most people who achieve ketosis report improvements in their sleep quality. However, initially this may not be the case. A common complaint and a sign you are in an early state of ketosis is that sleep is less than par. Not all people experience this, but some do – so if you do, stay the course. The good news is that it too is short-term, and once you are well into

ketosis, you will sleep like a baby.

If you want measurable proof that you're in ketosis, then you have to measure your ketones, which we'll discuss in depth in the next chapter!

Chapter 17. Am I In Ketosis? Tracking and Measuring Ketones

When following the Ketogenic Key methods to achieve ketosis, your body *will* produce ketone bodies, or you will be elevating your blood ketones through supplementation. There are three types of ketone bodies: acetone, acetoacetate, and beta-hydroxybutyrate (BHB). As mentioned above, ketone bodies can be measured through your breath, urine or blood. You can buy most of these tests at your local pharmacy, making it convenient and easy to measure your ketone levels at home.

There are several key signs and symptoms that can help you identify whether you are in nutritional ketosis without a test. If you are following the guidelines of the Ketogenic Key, and you are consistent, you will absolutely get into ketosis.

However, these signs may not be enough for you and you may want more of an accurate assessment, particularly in the beginning. This means monitoring either your blood, urine or breath.

What Are The Optimal Ketone Levels?

The Figure below shows the zones as defined by ketosis pioneers, Drs. Steven Phinney and Jeffery Volek.

0.5 – 3.0 (mmol/L) is considered the Optimal Ketone zone.

This is when ketones are plentiful enough to be utilized most effectively as energy by the brain, but also to fuel muscles and other organs. When ketone levels exceed 0.5 mmol/L, that's considered to be in a state of "ketosis."

3.0 – 10.0 (mmol/L) is considered the Starvation Ketosis zone.

It's important to note that when you get to this zone by following a ketogenic diet or supplementing with ketones, **this does not mean**

that you are actually starving. It means that you've achieved a level of ketosis where your body "thinks" it's starving because you've dropped your carbohydrate levels very low and your ketone levels are at an elevated level. When you are in this zone, fat is being metabolized and converted into ketones at a higher rate. This happens in a scenario like fasting and eating a high fat and very low carbohydrate diet on a consistent basis. This is a deeper ketotic state that will result in weight loss, deeper cellular autophagy, and is considered a therapeutic zone for conditions such as epilepsy and more.

10.0 mmol/L and over is considered a danger zone.

Elevated ketones past this level can move you into a toxic and potentially life-threatening state called diabetic ketoacidosis. But don't worry, you aren't going to get into this zone from following the diet or supplementing with ketones. Diabetic ketoacidosis is a dangerous condition in diabetics where their uncontrolled blood glucose elevates and stays elevated, but insulin is not shuttling it into the cells. They body senses that they aren't getting glucose in the cells, so it starts producing ketones. The glucose levels stay high, and yet the body keeps pumping out ketones. This combination of high ketones and elevated blood glucose creates a toxically acidic state in the body. If you are a diabetic, it is crucial that you track your blood ketone levels.

The Ketone Zone

Figure. From Volek JD and Phinney SD. The art and science of low-carbohydrate living: an expert guide to making the life-saving benefits of carbohydrate restriction sustainable and enjoyable. 2011; Lexington KY:Beyond Obesity.

Measuring your Ketones

Ketone Urine Strips

The simplest and least expensive method to measure your ketones is to use ketone urine testing strips, often referred to by the brand name Ketostix. The strips are inexpensive and help to check ketone levels quickly. Just as the name indicates, you pass the stick through your stream of urine and the strip will change its color to indicate the level of ketones in your urine. The keto strip changes color from its original beige — so you can compare the color to the guide on the package to find out how "deep" your level of ketosis is.

Deeper purple levels generally indicate higher levels of ketones. This doesn't mean deep levels are a desirable state though.

Be aware: ketone strips are the least accurate method to determine or measure ketosis. Drinking water can dilute the reading of ketones, equaling a false negative, and mild dehydration (such as first thing in the morning) can result in a false positive or higher than actual reading. In addition, when you use urine ketone strips, you are measuring the amount of ketones your body is excreting – or unused ketones. It does not indicate how high your blood ketone levels are, so this can sometime be misleading for assessing ketosis. In addition, if your body is very efficient at using ketones, there won't be as many being excreted in your urine. Therefore, sometimes a low reading does not mean you aren't in ketosis.

The Breath Analyzer Method

Hate peeing on ketone sticks, or want a more accurate test? Measuring your ketones can be as easy as breathing. The ketones in your breath are not the same as the ketones measured in blood. Breath ketones are a real-time indicator of using fat as fuel, which is a huge advantage when compared to measuring urine ketones.

Breath ketone analyzers are fairly accurate tools that measure the ketone acetone, which exits the body when you are in ketosis. Acetone is one of three ketone bodies (acetone, acetoacetate, and beta-hydroxybutyrate or BHB) produced by your body while in ketosis and used as energy.

Blood Testing For Ketones

If you are not averse to pricking your finger multiple times a week, at-home blood testing with a hand-held device is for you and is the most accurate because it measures the most predominant ketone in the body, beta-hydroxybutyrate (BHB) in your blood stream, so you are truly measuring the circulating ketone levels in your body. This form of testing also removes factors that can alter the results, such as how drinking water can dilute urine results or the effects of dehydration.

We recommend that you go by how you are feeling once you have verified that you are in ketosis. If you feel great, it is our opinion that you do not have to over-focus on your ketone levels. Many times, there are some whose bodies are so efficient at using ketones that they may not register via urine. So keep that in mind for those of you using the Ketogenic Key plan. Also, some people's bodies are very adept at burning fat and really do not require the amount of ketones comparatively. Many people who have been in long term ketosis can get by quite nicely on 20-30 net grams of carbs a day and might only show 0.4 to 0.7 millimolar (mmol/L) ketones on a blood test, but they have plenty of energy from burning free fatty acids and maintain muscle mass on relatively fewer calories than when they were dependent on carbs. Ultimately, how you feel physically and mentally should be your guide. But there are some reasons you might want to know where you fall in terms of your blood ketone levels, especially if you're diabetic.

Chapter 18. What Might Go Haywire? Things That Can Stall Keto Progress

Keto is not fool-proof and there are some things that may impede your progress. Let's say you are using the Ketogenic Key plan and you are not seeing any weight loss or belly shrinkage as quickly as you expected. Each body is different and responds differently to foods and other lifestyle choices. However, there may be very specific reasons why you are struggling to achieve your goals.

We have seen firsthand how this beneficial lifestyle can fail to yield results due to just a few simple unintentional mistakes, as well as thing that may simply be out of your control. Please note, many of the things below relate to weight loss, since that is the most common reason people choose to pursue the ketogenic diet or ketogenic therapies. Of course, there are MANY other health benefits to a keto lifestyle, and many of you reading this may be looking to simply improve your energy levels, enjoy a higher level of mental clarity and focus, or help quell low-level chronic inflammation. The good news is that the Ketogenic Key plan can help with all these things. But there are some common pitfalls and progress-stallers, which we want to address:

1. **Not Giving It Enough Time.**

    This may sound overly simplistic and obvious, but it merits some discussion, because it's easy to make mistakes – even unintentional ones – and lose interest and motivation if you don't see immediate results. Many people will take a cursory glance at the information in this book, and will believe they have all the information necessary and downloaded. They will hop on the plan and then, 10 days later, maybe they made some progress initially and then they hit a plateau, or they find they aren't deep in ketosis yet, their belly isn't shrinking or other goals aren't being met. Very important note: when it comes to following the Ketogenic Key recommendations, you must be patient, and give your body time to transition to a new way of fueling itself!

When adjusting to a ketogenic diet, the first rule initially is to bring your carb intake down. Most proponents of a well-formulated ketogenic diet recommend reducing your intake to 25 grams of carbohydrates per day, maybe even less. This is why it's important to track your carb intake, and it's also important to track your ketone levels so that you know whether you're getting into ketosis or not. It's just as important to give yourself TIME – give yourself at least 2 weeks to adjust to this new way of fueling your body. After a couple of weeks, if you are not getting into ketosis, you may need to reduce your carb intake a bit lower, or you may need to combine diet with one or more of the other methods we describe (supplementation, intermittent fasting, and exercise).

If your goal is weight loss, patience is key. In the beginning, most people lose a lot of weight and then it slows or tapers off and they think it's not working. They might initially lose up to a pound a day, and if it slows to a pound a week or even stays at the same weight, they become frustrated. But rest assured that your Ketogenic Key lifestyle is working. As a rule of thumb, the most weight a healthy person should lose is between 1 and 2 pounds per week. That fat didn't appear on your body overnight, and it won't leave overnight. It's going to take some time. The goal of the Ketogenic Key is to help you become metabolically flexible and healthy, and eventually the weight will come off. Focus on the other indicators in the meantime, such as: energy level, sleep quality, memory, focus, and reduced or reversed inflammation. Keep your attention on those, not just the weight loss. Don't give up if you are only losing one-half to one-pound a week. Just tweak what you are doing. Remember, if you are exercising, you may be building some muscle, which is healthy, but may counter the loss of fat weight. Let the mirror and how your clothes fit be indicators of your success!

2.   Having an Unusually Slow Metabolism

If you are having a hard time losing fat on the diet, it may be that your metabolism is really slow. Maybe this is due to the fact that, if you're a middle-aged woman, going through menopause is slowing it down. Or maybe you have been on and off yo-yo diets in the past, which have caused you to develop a slower metabolism. If so, you might have to bring your carb intake down, maybe as low as 10 grams per day – this is what is necessary to counter that slow metabolism. We also suggest that you have a moderate amount of protein (6 ounces of protein at each meal), a large quantity of vegetables, and that you consume enough fat to satiate your hunger from one meal to the next. This is a key concept. You need to stay satiated while you are transitioning from glucose dependence (carbohydrates) to utilizing fat and ketones for energy.

3.   Overeating Fat and/or Calories

For those of you targeting fat loss as a goal (as opposed to other benefits), as you begin to see success and get into the diet more, it's important to ensure that you're not overeating fat and/or calories, because what we don't want is your body to only turn the dietary fat into ketones and not your own body fat into ketones. This is an instance where we would strongly recommend tracking macros and calories with a tool like MyFitnessPal. Because if you are trying to lose weight and fat, you need to be sure you're in a calorie deficit along with getting into ketosis, so your body has no choice but to start burning those body fat stores for energy!

Because fat is so calorie-dense, it's easy to over consume fat and calories. For example, it's easy to add too much fat into foods during cooking, if you go heavy on oils and butter. Measuring how much butter and oil is a good idea, especially at the start, until you get a feel for being able to "eyeball" the amount. Another easy thing to overeat is nuts or nut butters. A typical serving size is about a handful of nuts, but in our snacking culture it's easy to have 3 or 4 times that because they are small. But nuts are very calorie-dense, so a little goes a long way!

The other Key is exercise and activity – to ensure that you are getting enough activity in your day and managing your calorie intake to create an energy deficit – in other words, you want to be burning more calories per day than you eat in food. This doesn't mean you have to be a gym rat. It just means you should balance your activity level and amount of calories consumed (using a tool like MyFitnessPal) so that you burn more calories than you eat – that way you ensure your body is tapping into your body fat for energy, not just the foods you are eating.

4.   Not Employing Intermittent Fasting.

One way to take the express train to ketosis is to incorporate intermittent fasting into your routine while you are eating a very low carb/keto diet and/or supplementing with exogenous ketones. Fasting ensures your body has to tap into your fat stores for energy (as mentioned above), and when you do it intermittently, you protect your metabolism from slowing down.

Not choosing to do intermittent fasting when your goal is weight loss is like trying to run a marathon on your knees. By doing intermittent fasting you can greatly accelerate the results by markedly decreasing your insulin response. As we noted earlier in the book, insulin is a hormone that signals your body to store calories as fat. This combination of a very low carbohydrate diet and intermittent fasting for stubborn weight or stubborn belly fat is, in our opinion, an excellent recipe for success. Additionally, there are many therapeutic health reasons why you would want to add it to your optimal health regime. Check out the Intermittent Fasting chapter for more details and direction.

5.   Having Non-Alcoholic Fatty Liver Disease

Many obese or overweight people have a condition called non-alcoholic fatty liver disease (NAFLD). In fact, it's estimated that between 10 and 20% of American have it. NAFLD is characterized by fat buildup in and around the liver, which is due to the liver processing large amounts of sugar, high-fructose corn syrup, and refined carbohydrates that are prevalent in the standard American diet. The good news is that it is reversible, and if treated early, doesn't cause damage to the liver. The problem is that having a non-alcoholic fatty liver impedes its crucial functions (like clearing toxins), fat metabolism and reduces your body's capacity to make ketones and growth hormone. As we noted before, ketones are created in the liver by metabolizing fatty acids. So it's important to try to reverse NAFLD if you have it, and get one of the most crucial organs in your body back to optimal performance!

Weight loss (specifically fat loss) is the most effective method to reverse NAFLD. Following the Ketogenic Key plan and using intermittent fasting along with a supplement called choline, can help metabolize the fat in and around the liver. Some people see significant improvements after about 6 weeks of fat loss. Just bear in mind that the body will have to remove the fat in and around the liver and other organs (visceral fat) first, before the fat in the abdomen can shrink. Patience is key in this instance, because it will take some time for that visceral fat to de-accumulate. But getting rid of that visceral fat, and reversing fatty liver disease is a very important component to optimizing your overall health. If you have NAFLD and are having a hard time losing weight, over time following the Ketogenic Key plan you will lose weight, and this will help reverse your fatty liver and in turn, weight loss and ketosis will start coming easier!

6. Gaining Muscle Mass (actually this is a good thing!)

Many people who have been sedentary and begin exercising initially gain a little weight because as they are losing fat, they are also gaining muscle (don't worry, you won't gain big muscles and look like Arnold Schwarzenegger!). And because muscle is more dense than fat, a little muscle can add weight to your body even as you're losing fat. If you are trying to only judge your progress by your weight on a scale, this may be discouraging. This is why we encourage people to not worry about scale weight, and focus on how they feel, how they look in the mirror, and how their clothes fit. The scale tells you very little about health improvements. So if you initially gain a little scale weight, don't panic! You may just be replacing some of that atrophied muscle while your body composition is changing and fat is being burned.

The other reason we say gaining muscle is a good thing, is that having healthy muscle on your body optimizes your metabolism. Muscle requires energy to maintain and use, so having it helps you burn more calories! In fact, gaining muscle can actually accelerate your fat loss.

If you are female and menopausal, chances are higher you have more atrophied muscle mass, essentially a loss of muscle that occurs naturally as we age starting in our 30s but accelerating after menopause because of hormonal changes. Strength training is *crucial* to help promote weight loss, and is very effective. It doesn't happen overnight but know changes are taking place. Plan to strength train with weights or use body weight training exercises such as push-ups, body-weight squats, pull-ups etc. Which brings us to our next point...

7.   Not Exercising or Being Active Enough

Exercise is not the top choice to help you lose weight – diet is. You've probably heard things like "weight loss is 80% diet, 20% exercise." Or that "abs are built in the kitchen, not in the gym." These statements are true. That being said, exercise is a very important aspect of overall health. Combining exercise and activity with a very low-carb/keto diet is a powerful and effective method to rid one of stubborn fat, partly due to exercise's ability to burn calories, stimulate growth hormone and boost metabolism.

As mentioned previously, it's key to create an energy deficit – to expend more calories than you are eating, so that your body is forced to tap into its fat stores to supply energy by converting that fat to ketone bodies. You don't have to do intense or prolonged exercise sessions to do this. Even something as simple as walking every day can help you burn more calories. Simple things like parking at the far end of the parking lot and taking stairs instead of elevators or escalators can help you burn calories and create that magical energy deficit!

Chapter 18. What Might Go Haywire?

If you are exercising, we suggest trying high intensity interval training (HIIT) or short little bursts of effort to maximize your metabolic rate and supercharge your fat loss efforts. Refer to our exercise section for guidance.

8.   Stress and Lack of Sleep

Stress and lack of sleep can severely limit your ability to lose weight and can suppress the keto benefits of increased energy and mental focus and clarity. A myriad of things can cause stress and therefore, for many, lack of sleep. Lack of sleep means more stress and vice versa. In both cases, the hormone cortisol is generated. This hormone is highly beneficial for weight loss and other bodily functions, but when it is too high for too long or suppressed, either of which can happen due to stress and lack of sleep, it can become exactly the opposite and be detrimental to your weight loss efforts and overall health. Therefore, it is important to address any sleep issues or stress issues that arise. If you struggle with sleep and stress, practice stress relief and positive sleep habits that will enable you to experience quality sleep and reduced stress, and keep your cortisol at beneficial levels.

Chapter 19. Keto Flu: What Is It, and How To Manage It

When embarking upon the ketogenic diet, or any very low-carb protocol, there are some people who experience what is called the "keto flu," a physical state that has a variety of flu-like symptoms. These symptoms can lead an inexperienced keto dieter to believe the diet isn't working for them, or that they are getting sick because of it. Thankfully, that's not the case at all! Keto flu is a natural response to the shock of changing your body's fuel source from glucose to ketones, and it's important to note that it's only temporary, and it can be prevented, mitigated and/or reversed.

What symptoms are typical during the keto flu? It presents with things such as:

- Fatigue
- Sugar Cravings
- Difficulty Focusing
- Dizziness
- Irritability
- Insomnia
- Digestive upset

Interestingly, most of these symptoms are exactly the opposite of what you will experience once you get through keto flu and enter the state of ketosis! The good news is that if you get it, it happens quickly and doesn't last long. Generally, those who experience the keto flu will do so within the first week of cutting back carbohydrates in their diet.

So, why does the keto flu develop? Well, it's really quite logical. In most people, their body has been dependent upon carbohydrates (glucose) for fuel for their entire life (at least since they stopped breastfeeding as a baby and started being fed fruit, carbohydrates, and sugar). If that glucose or carb intake is reduced substantially, as it is with the ketogenic diet, your body is depleted of stored glucose and instead turns to burning fatty acids (fat) for energy.

160

Chapter 18. What Might Go Haywire?

This is the metabolic process of *ketosis.* The keto flu is a natural reaction when our bodies are entering ketosis and switching from a state of glucose-burning to fat-burning – this is what we desire, to be able to burn fat stores and reap the myriad health benefits of ketosis too! But there is typically a transition period where the body is depleted of carbohydrates and glucose, but hasn't ramped up the production of ketone bodies yet, and this can cause fatigue and other symptoms typically associated with keto flu.

How long does it last?

It varies from person to person. Typically about 3 days to 1 week, with some reporting symptoms into the second week. Again, this is atypical, noting that *most individuals do not experience this* and if the keto flu does occur, it is very short-lived. The good news is that there are things you can do to lessen the likelihood of experiencing these symptoms, or to mitigate them quickly if they do occur.

How to Prevent and/or Get Rid of The Keto "Flu"

Ease Into it

One way to avoid the keto flu is to avoid an overnight change from eating a standard American diet high in carbs, to going almost zero carb. Cut back your carbs gradually over a couple of weeks, so that your body begins to transition slowly, and you'll almost assuredly avoid the keto flu.

Stay Hydrated

Drinking water is very important because need to replenish the vast amount of water lost during the initial launch into the ketogenic diet. Being in ketosis can cause your body to require higher amounts of water to stay hydrated, and so being dehydrated alone can cause the keto flu. Try to drink up to one gallon (128 ounces) of water a day. Clear urine is a sign you are adequately hydrated. Keep your water bottle or bottles filled-up and around you all day. This will have far-reaching effects upon your health and weight.

Replenish Electrolytes

What are electrolytes? Think calcium, potassium, magnesium, and sea salt. Without electrolytes, our cells would die-off or burst from being too full. An electrolyte imbalance can cause or exacerbate keto flu symptoms. Stay ahead of the game by increasing your salt intake with a pinch of pink Himalayan salt in your water, drink bone broth that is high in potassium and sodium, and consider hydrating and supplementing with a bio-available form of magnesium.

Get Your Sleep

Your body is experiencing a lot of changes as it switches fuel sources, so getting plenty of sleep can help reduce stress and fatigue. Take a short nap during the day, if necessary.

Go Easy On Exercise

If you are jumping into keto cold turkey, you will likely feel depleted your first week. Try to do some light exercise rather than going all out in your exercise program. Go for walks or other fairly non-intensive activities. Then, when your energy levels resume, increase your activity level. This will help you to switch between using carbs as your sole energy source to using your fat for fuel. When you do this, you are helping to prevent or mitigate the keto flu.

Increase Your Consumption of Fats and Proteins

When you cut carbs to a low enough level to be considered "ketogenic," your body will no longer be getting energy from carbohydrates and sugars, and it takes time to transition to the point that it can tap into your body's fat stores for energy (becoming fat-adapted or keto-adapted). So it needs plenty of fat for fuel from your diet. But if there isn't enough dietary fat, it can't find the energy it needs, which can contribute to the keto flu symptoms. Make sure that you replace the carbs with healthy fats and quality proteins.

Supplement With Exogenous Ketones

In the past few years, supplemental ketone products have hit the market. The ones that contain the ketone body beta-

Chapter 18. What Might Go Haywire?

hydroxybutyrate (BHB) can be very beneficial in making the transition from being a glucose-burner to a fat and ketone burner, and increasing the level of ketones circulating in your body. When you eliminate carbs from your diet, you are eliminating the fuel your body is accustomed to burning, and so providing ketones directly into your system to use as fuel can help avoid the side effects of keto flu as your body adjusts to the diet. Ketone bodies are a high-yield fuel, providing 38% more ATP (energy for your cells) than glucose. So supplementing with them can give your body the fuel it needs to run efficiently. Both of the authors use and recommend daily ketone supplementation for a number of reasons, which are covered in more detail in the supplementation chapter in this book.

If you do experience some of the keto flu symptoms, follow the above protocol and they will subside.

Chapter 20. Keto-Adaption and Exercise Performance

As we have discussed in the book so far, in order to get into the healthful state of ketosis we are aiming for with the Ketogenic Key lifestyle, one has to go through a period of adaptation – and to do that, one must either (a) severely restrict carbohydrate intake, (b) practice fasting, (c) exercise enough to burn glucose stores, or all three! In this section, we want to discuss exercise and general activity as a way to achieve, enhance, and complement being in a state of ketosis, and talk about some of the challenges you can face when you initially start exercising during keto-adaptation – and how to overcome those challenges!

History shows that we humans are genetically wired to be able to move our bodies without food availability for periods of time, and with very little intake of dietary carbohydrates. Some of the best examples can be seen historically from hunter/gatherers, and more recently from the Inuit people. The traditional Inuit diet was largely devoid of carbohydrates and essentially fat and protein (meat) focused. They were hunters, and prolonged movement was necessary for their survival. They did just fine without carbohydrates, and so will you!

Eating a very low carbohydrate ketogenic diet is a healthful choice and doable for all levels of fitness.

As we have mentioned before, the human body is capable of using different fuel sources. The most common source is glucose, due to most people eating a standard American diet that is high in sugar and starchy carbohydrates, which convert quickly into blood glucose to fuel the body and brain. Fats can also be broken down to fatty acids and glycerol to use as energy and help the body use glucose as a fuel, although this is not the most efficient and high-output source of energy for our bodies. However, when we achieve a state of ketosis, our bodies convert our own body fat or dietary fat into ketones, which are like rocket fuel for your body and reign supreme over the other sources of fuel like glucose. Ketones

Chapter 20. Keto-Adaption and Exercise Performance

generate 38% more adenosine triphosphate (ATP), which is what your cells' mitochondria use for fuel. That's a big difference!

Adapting to utilizing ketones for fuel, when we have been dependent on glucose our whole lives, can take time and can be different for everyone. Generally however, when one is just starting the ketogenic diet, it may take up to two weeks to become keto-adapted, and for some folks it can even take up to a couple of months.

A few of the most common question we get is "Should I work out, or avoid working out, when starting keto or any very low carbohydrate diet?" "Will it affect my performance?" and "What type of workout should I do when in ketosis?" The short answers are (1) yes, it's very possible to workout on keto without experiencing a loss of physical performance, and (2) different types of workouts can both benefit from and complement the state of ketosis. Think of ketosis and working out as being synergistic.

Most people are aware that carbohydrates provide energy to get through a workout, and going on a ketogenic diet severely restricts carbohydrates...so now what? How is your body going to sail through a workout without its normal fuel? Fear not! The good news is that your body is capable of using your own fat for its energy demands. Having said that, your workouts may be challenging until after you have adapted to your new way of eating. **The performance benefits of keto take a few weeks to manifest as your body switches from using glucose to fat (converted to ketones) for fuel, and during this time, a common side effect of the keto transition is *reduced* performance in the gym. However, there are ways to counter this problem. One of them is to supplement with exogenous ketones while you are going through this keto-adaption period, so that your body has extra fuel to run on. For many people, it helps them through that adaption period.**

However, after a while you will find the opposite may begin to happen. Once you've been on a keto diet or other very low-carb diet for at least a few weeks, you should be in an extended state of ketosis, and your body should be burning fat instead of glucose. As we mentioned previously, fat has more calories (energy) per gram than glucose or protein, and ketones also generate about 38% more

ATP than glucose does. Therefore, keto actually increases energy efficiency. You may find that you perform better than before when working out – more endurance, less lactic acid burn, and not getting out of breath as easily. You may even find that your intensity gets jacked up, because the more your body is able to utilize fat for ongoing fueling, the more glycogen (glucose) you preserve for truly intense efforts.

Maintaining Energy and Athletic/Fitness Performance During the Transition

In order to ensure that you keep your energy levels high while your body adapts to the keto lifestyle, there are a few things to keep in mind:

Increase Your Fat Consumption

During the transition period of approximately 2 weeks, increase your intake of fat. Yes, you will be doing this naturally on the ketogenic diet, but for the first 2 weeks, add in a bit more. This will upregulate your energy producing mitochondria to help burn fat and the important AMPK (5 adenosine monophosphate-activated protein kinase) enzyme. AMPK plays a major role in cellular energy, activating fatty acid uptake when your energy is low. The extra addition of that fat will also speed up your body's ability to utilize ketones for fuel.

Have an extra handful or two of macadamia nuts or other nuts like almonds, a bit more extra virgin olive oil or avocado oil, add in a few fatty snacks such as coconut flakes or hard-boiled eggs. Also, add in fish high in omega 3 fats that will increase your AMPK such as wild salmon, sardines or mackerel.

Add In Minerals and Electrolytes

Whether you are exercising or not, minerals count! When you are on the ketogenic diet, you will lose a lot of water and the minerals go right out with it. This is why it is vital to add minerals and electrolytes: to not only prevent the "keto flu," but to keep you energized, hydrated, motivated and active.

Chapter 22. Ketogenic Key Foods:

Always experiment to find what works best for you, but here is what works in general for most people: about 2 teaspoons (4.5 grams) of fine sea salt or a little under 3 teaspoons of kosher salt (not regular table salt), sprinkled in food. Also, add a couple of pinches in drinking water. Use 300-400 mg of magnesium, and 1-2 grams of potassium each day on top of your normal food or as a supplement. Again, the salt you can easily add to your water or other drinks, and that will help restore your sodium level while working out.

Use Creatine

Creatine has the powerful ability to increase your body's stores of phosphocreatine, which your body can use to generate large amounts of ATP or energy for quick bursts of high-intensity exercise or heavy lifting. The added natural energy is going to help assist in your fitness efforts, meaning you will have more energy available to exercise. This will improve your overall performance and results.

Creatine also prevents muscle loss and adds muscle mass. Keto and creatine go very well together. You can take it at any time – simply mix it with any liquid such as water, coffee or a protein shake.

We do not recommend you use creatine if you have pre-existing kidney or liver problems. That said, creatine has a well-researched safety profile and is one of the most researched supplements to date. Recent studies showed that creatine did not have any negative effects on healthy people with normal liver and kidney function.

Use Exogenous Ketones

As discussed earlier in the book, exogenous ketone supplements (racemic ketone salts or ketone monoesters) are somewhat new and are rapidly growing in popularity. New research is increasingly showing them to have excellent potential health benefits. They can be incredibly helpful as an adjunct to a keto diet, or as a way to bridge the gap between a normal low-carb diet and achieving blood ketone levels equivalent to or even higher than nutritional ketosis. When we have ketones in our body, whether exogenously or through our diet, ketones are glycogen sparing, which means that we will be able to readily use that glycogen in our muscles that is constantly being stored, and utilize it for energy demands like workouts or bursts of activity.

Managing Your Workouts During the Keto-Adaptation Period

During the initial keto-adaptation transition, if you feel like you are struggling during your normal workouts, you may need to take it easier than you normally would for a while. If your body is not yet well adapted to utilizing its fat stores, it may be difficult to have the intensity you are used to having. We would not recommend you run your first triathlon or even a 5k when you are first delving into the ketogenic diet. However, once you are in ketosis and fat-adapted, you may find that cardio and endurance exercise becomes significantly easier! Many ultramarathon competitors are converts to the keto lifestyle because of the increased energy benefit of burning fat and ketones.

Once you're fully fat-adapted and able to utilize fats, ketones, and glycogen, you're going to be unstoppable in the gym – as well as at home, at work, and everywhere!!

"When you train on your newly keto diet, think of it like you're increasing weight, upping the intensity, or learning a new sport. You're not weaker. You're not getting worse. The training is getting harder. The pain is increasing. And, although it might not feel like it right now, you're going to be better off in the long run."
~Mark Sisson

Ketosis Helps You Maximize Your Exercise!

The health benefits of exercising become enhanced while in ketosis. Whether interval training, resistance training, or simply walking long-distance – the results will be enhanced.

First and foremost, you'll burn more fat! Research shows that during a long run, keto-adapted athletes saw 2 to 3 times more fat oxidation occurred and muscle glycogen was replenished similarly. Compared to highly trained ultra-endurance athletes consuming a

Chapter 22. Ketogenic Key Foods:

high-carb diet, the athletes who were in long-term keto-adaptation experienced extraordinarily high rates of fat oxidation.

Next, being in ketosis helps to prevent fatigue during exercise – a common experience for many when working out or competing in athletic events. There are a few reasons for this. First of all, as we've mentioned before, ketones generate more ATP. Second, exercise physiology studies have shown that athletes in ketosis experience lower levels of lactic acid build-up (this is the thing that causes what is called "the burn" where the muscles begin to have a burning sensation and tire out). Third, blood sugar stabilization helps to maintain and promote a powerful workout because the body is metabolically balanced. Finally, there is a brain component to working out, and ketones help the brain operate at peak efficiency, so athletes who are in ketosis report laser-like mental focus and acuity. Research provides evidence that when you are keto-adapted, pretty much all forms of exercise will be much more effective, and your body and brain will perform at a higher level.

Chapter 21. Types of Exercise: Maximizing Your Ketogenic Key Lifestyle

So now that you are following the Ketogenic Key lifestyle, and experiencing the benefits of ketosis, your next question may be "what type of exercise should I do?"

The truth is that any exercise is an excellent choice. However, as mentioned previously, depending upon where you are in the transition, this may dictate your choice. Keep in mind that exercise itself can induce ketosis as a result of the mobilization of fatty acids to the liver where they are essentially broken down into ketone bodies. Generally, exercise puts us in a state of ketosis, just not a dietary state of ketosis. Let's just say ketones combined with cardio create a very clean cellular environment vs eating a lot of carbohydrates and doing cardio produces a lot of cellular waste or what we call "dirty energy" which includes an enormous amount of reactive oxygen species (ROS).

There are four different types of exercises to choose from and all are important to optimal health and fitness in different ways:

1. Aerobic
2. Anaerobic
3. Plyometric
4. Flexibility/stability

And as the intensity of the exercise increases, the body changes what it uses as its source of fuel. Exercise intensity alters the metabolism of nutritional ketosis.

Ketones can only be burned in the mitochondria, which are the tiny organelles that are the power or energy plants of every cell. So that means that ketones cannot be used as much as an anaerobic source of energy.

In one study, high performance athletes endured one hour of intense cycling. Before the exercise, they were given either a ketone ester drink (exogenous ketones), or a carbohydrate drink, or they gave them a fatty acid drink. Interestingly, the ketone ester group ended up having lower levels of plasma glucose, lower levels of lactic acid and lower levels of free fatty acids, which goes to show they were using ketones instead of glucose. They were sparing the glycogen – meaning that ketones are glycogen sparing.

What does this mean? Ketosis increases metabolic flexibility during exercise – allowing the body to use either glycogen (glucose) or fat (ketones) for fuel, and increases muscle fat oxidation. The athletes' improved performance while in ketosis shows us that being in ketosis during exercise is beneficial.

Let's break down the different forms of exercise that are excellent to use when in ketosis.

Aerobic Exercises

Aerobic exercise is what we typically refer to as "cardio' and is an excellent choice when you are on a ketogenic diet or in ketosis from intermittent fasting or supplementation, and trying to lose fat. The textbook distinction between aerobic and anaerobic exercise is whether or not oxygen is used to produce the energy required for the effort.

Even cardio exercises that are low-intensity and fat-burning still rely upon oxygen to produce energy. Examples of aerobic exercise include sessions on a bike, treadmill, elliptical, running, and even brisk walks.

Anaerobic Exercises

Very low carbohydrate diets are excellent without compromise to muscle mass or function. And when your body is in ketosis, the anaerobic system does not react to exercise as it does in an aerobic system. This is because your body requires energy from the anaerobic system for short-term high-intensity exercise.

The anaerobic system relies on glycolysis, or the breakdown of glucose for energy. Because a very low carb way of eating requires your body to use fat for energy instead of glucose, it basically has an empty tank for quick burst energy exercise. So you may find that consuming carbs right before this sort of exercise is beneficial to maintaining intensity (don't worry, you will burn them off!).

Examples of anaerobic exercise include **high intensity interval training (HIIT)**, plyometric exercises and strength training. A basic example of a HIIT workout on any machine, or with walking, running or even using your own bodyweight:

- 30 Seconds All Out (High Intensity)
- 90 Seconds Slow to Moderate Pace
- Repeat 8 Times

That's it! There are different protocols and time variations, but the common theme in HIIT is that you do a period of super high intensity, followed by a longer period of recover at a lower intensity – but you don't specifically rest. This keeps your body burning calories and oxidizing fat at a high rate!

HIIT has been shown to have numerous health benefits in addition to the fact that it burns fat at a high level. One such benefit is improved cognitive function.

Plyometric Exercises

Plyometric Exercises are anaerobic and improve muscle strength, speed, endurance and fat loss. Plyometric are exercises that involve jumping or explosive movement. For example, skipping, bounding, jumping rope, hopping, lunges or jump squats are all plyometric exercises. Jumping rope is a low-level plyometric exercise and is great for beginners. And with practice and increased intensity of the *jumps* performed, *rope jumping* can even become a high-level *plyometric exercise.*

Very low carbohydrate diets such as the ketogenic diet, generally do not contribute to a loss in performance with plyometric exercises.

Flexibility Exercises

Stretching our muscles leads to a flexible body and this is important to overall fitness, a better workout, and faster recovery.

Major stretching benefits include:
- Increased movement efficiency
- Decreased risk of injury
- Increased circulation and nutrients to muscles and joint structures
- Increased neuromuscular coordination
- Decreased risk of low back pain
- Reduced muscular tension
- Improved balance and postural awareness

There are countless stretching exercises (just do a Google or YouTube search and see!), and we recommend that everyone, regardless of activity level, should engage in stretching.

Stability Exercises

Stability is an often-overlooked part of optimized fitness. Adding this important component to your exercise regimen will pay huge rewards.

According to the American Council on Exercise (ACE), stability is defined as the ability to maintain control of joint movement or position by coordinating actions of surrounding tissues and the neuromuscular system.

These types of exercises are what we use to train our core, and they improve our ability to balance. This aids us in proper alignment, movement control, and muscle strength, leading to what we call "balance." Even if stability comes naturally, we can all continually improve upon it.

Examples of stability exercises:

- Incorporate unilateral exercises (one arm or one leg at a time) or by changing your stance.

- Planks – all varieties
- Lunges – all varieties
- Squats – all varieties
- Yoga
- Balance or Wobble Boards
- BOSU Balls
- Exercise Balls

Want more ideas? Search YouTube for videos on improving stability and core strength!

In summary, following a ketogenic diet and/or supplementing with exogenous ketone supplements can have a significant impact on your health, fitness, and sport or competitive pursuits. Just remember, it may take your body some time to adapt to the diet, if you choose to go that route, and any initial challenges you have with fatigue or lack of energy will soon resolve. Once that happens, and your body is being fueled by ketones, you'll feel and perform like a different person – a better version of you!

Section VI: What to Eat and What Not to Eat, Shopping Lists, and Recipes

Part I. Food and Drink

Some of the most frequent questions we get when talking to people about healthy eating and keto friendly meals is, "Do you have any recipes you can share?" Or, "What do you actually EAT on a keto diet?" So we thought we'd make it easy for you and include some food lists and guidance on what to eat, and what not to eat, address questions about alcohol and fiber, and provide you with a bunch of recipes that take the guess work out of making delicious meals and snacks.

Chapter 22. Ketogenic Key Foods: What to Eat – What Not to Eat

An eating plan doesn't have to be frustrating or complex. One of the best features of the Ketogenic Key lifestyle is that it is simple. Keto works because it changes the very "fuel source" that the body uses to stay energized: namely, from burning glucose (or sugar) to dietary or stored fat due to the types of foods used.

What food(s) trigger ketosis? Is it fat, protein or carbohydrates? A lot of times people associate a high fat or high protein diet with ketosis, this is not the thing that puts us in ketosis. Rather, it is the absence of glucose in the diet that triggers the production of ketones.

If you're aiming to achieve nutritional ketosis, your keto meal plan should contain high amounts of healthy fats (at least 70% and up to 80 % of your total calories), such as olive oil, coconut oil, MCT oil, grass-fed butter, fatty meats and fish, and some nuts and seeds. Fats are a critical part of every recipe because fat is what provides not only energy, but also prevents hunger, weakness and fatigue.

The veggies on a keto plate should be mostly non-starchy vegetables such as: broccoli and other cruciferous veggies, all types of leafy greens, asparagus, cucumber, and zucchini. Vegetables are counted as carbohydrates; however, with the Ketogenic Key plan, you will be counting "net carbs" - not total carbs.

How to Calculate Net Carbs on Keto — and Why They Matter

Should you care about net carbs? Well yes. If you are on a low carb diet, it is important that you know what "net carbs" are and how to calculate them.

Net carbs are the carbohydrates in food that you can digest and use for energy. Net carbs are calculated by taking your total grams of carbs and subtract out grams of fiber. That results in your net carbs.

Fiber = Net Carbs

if a food has 12 grams of carbs and 6 grams of fiber, subtract the fiber from the carbohydrate total (12 – 6 = 6) and you will have a net carb total of 6 grams. Use the net carbs in your total carb count. To truly optimize nutritional ketosis, the most important point to remember is to eat no more than 20 grams of net carbohydrates per day. Now, it is possible to achieve ketosis by eating as many as 50 grams per day (a number that is thrown around a lot as a "target" for grams of carbs per day), but it's likely that you will not be very deep into ketosis and may or may not be able to sustain ketosis at that level.

Ketogenic Key Food List

The percentages of macros on the keto diet look like this: 5% carbs, 70-80% fat and 15-20% protein. Easy right? Let's talk about the three macronutrients briefly, to make sure everything's clear and we keep it simple!

Proteins

Animal proteins (meat, fish, etc.) have very little, if any, carbs. You can consume them in moderate amounts as needed to control hunger. Overall, choose fattier cuts of meat rather than leaner ones. For example, chicken thighs and legs are considered darker meat and preferable to chicken breasts because they contain much more fat that will keep you satiated.

In moderation, you want high quality proteins, which are foods that contain the nine essential amino acids the body needs. Out of the 20 amino acids that are found in your body's proteins, 9 are essential to your diet because your cells cannot manufacture them

Without enough protein, your body will start using the muscle as a source of energy – even before your fat stores.

Your plate should reflect foods that are high in protein but low- or no-carb, including grass-fed meat, pasture-raised poultry, cage-free eggs, bone broth, wild-caught fish, organ meats and some full-fat (ideally raw) dairy products. Here are our recommendations for good keto proteins:

Grass-fed beef and other types of fatty cuts of meat (try to avoid antibiotics in all meats) including lamb, goat, veal, venison and other game. Grass-fed, fatty meat is preferable because it's higher in quality omega-3 fats.

Organ meats — most organ meats contain almost no carbs, except for liver, where glycogen is stored. Liver may contain around 3-5 grams net carbs per 5 ounces

Poultry, including turkey, chicken, quail, pheasant, hen, goose, duck — 0 grams net carbs per 5 ounces

Cage-free eggs and egg yolks — 0.5-gram carb each. (Including deviled, fried, scrambled and boiled — use the whole egg; the yolk is where all the fat is!)

Seafood, all varieties; including wild shellfish, wild fish: tuna, wild rainbow trout, anchovies, wild sea bass, wild flounder, wild mackerel, wild salmon, wild sardines, shrimp, clams, mussels, etc.

Nuts, nut butters and seeds (particularly nuts that are low in carbs such as pecans and macadamia nuts over nuts high in carbs like cashews and pistachios).

Protein powders (unsweetened). Note: if you use protein powders a lot, we recommend checking your blood glucose after eating them. In some cases, micronized protein can cause spikes in blood sugar, so it's good to verify if this is happening if you're trying to keep your blood glucose consistently stable.

Carbohydrates

All leafy greens, including dandelion or beet greens, collards, mustard, turnip, arugula, chicory, endive, escarole, fennel, radicchio, romaine, sorrel, spinach, kale, chard, etc. — range from 0.5–5 net carbs per 1 cup

Cruciferous veggies like broccoli, cabbage, Brussels sprouts and cauliflower — 3–6 grams net carbs per 1 cup

Celery, cucumber, zucchini, chives and leeks — 2–4 grams net carbs per 1 cup

Section VI

Certain fermented foods like sauerkraut, kimchi, and dairy or coconut kefir (also beneficial for gut health) — 1–2 grams net carbs per 1/2 cup (make sure there is no sugar added as sometimes happens with commercial preparations of sauerkraut and kimchi)

Fresh herbs - close to 0 grams net carbs per 1–2 tablespoons

Veggies that are slightly higher in carbs but still low include: asparagus, mushrooms, bamboo shoots, bean sprouts, bell pepper, sugar snap peas, water chestnuts, radishes, jicama, green beans, wax beans, tomatoes — 3–7 grams net carbs per 1 cup raw.

Starchy Carbs

We suggest you avoid these, or if you must eat them, eat in very small quantities or you will easily surpass your daily carb limit in one meal!

Acorn squash –14.9 grams net carbs per 1 cup
Sweet potato - 22 grams net carbs per 1 cup
Grains
Potatoes
Parsnips

*When considering whether grains have a place in your diet, you need to look at how many net carbs it contains (not total carbs). Grains low in net carbs include oatmeal, soba noodles, bulgur, buckwheat, whole-wheat pasta and wild rice. Eating foods low in net carbs ensures you will digest the carbohydrates more slowly while feeling full longer.

*The average person will mostly likely need to stay within 25-30 grams of net carbohydrates per day to stay in ketosis, and possibly 20 grams or less to stay in deep ketosis

Healthy Fats

Most healthy fats contain zero net carbohydrates. The fats listed below are exceptional as well for their health benefits. Healthy fats include saturated fats, monounsaturated fats and certain types of polyunsaturated fats (PUFAs), especially omega-3 fatty acids. It's best to include all types of fats in your daily regimen.

Cold-pressed coconut oil
MCT oil
MCT powder
Grass-fed butter
Ghee
Coconut butter
Mayonnaise (avocado based)
Palm fruit
Avocado oil
Walnut oil
Olive oil
Flaxseed oil
Sesame oil
Macadamia nut oil
Lard
Chicken fat
Duck fat
Avocado
Nuts
Seeds

Drinks

Water
Coffee or tea without added sugar (dairy is fine)
Bone broth
Broth

Keto Foods to Limit — Eat In Moderation To Stay In Ketosis

Full-Fat Dairy

Dairy products should be used strategically as the natural milk sugars or carbs can add-up quickly unless using as a condiment. Higher fat, hard cheeses have the least carbs, while low-fat milk and soft cheeses have much more.

- Full-fat cow's and goat milk (ideally organic and raw) — 11–12 net carb grams per one cup serving

Section VI

- Full Fat Yogurts (unsweetened)
- Full-fat cheeses — 0.5–1.5 net carb grams per one ounce or about 1/4 cup
- Full-fat cottage cheese — 5 net carb grams per 1/2 cup

Medium-Starchy Vegetables

- Sweet peas, artichokes, okra, carrots, beets and parsnips — about 7–14 net carb grams per 1/2 cup cooked
- Yams and potatoes (white, red, sweet, etc.) — sweet potatoes have the least carbs, about 10 net carb grams per 1/2 potato; yams and white potatoes can have much more, about 13–25 net carb grams per 1/2 potato/yam cooked

Legumes and Beans

- Garbanzo beans, kidney beans, lima beans, black beans, brown beans, lentils, hummus, etc. — about 12–13 net carb grams per 1/2 cup serving cooked
- Soy products, including tofu, edamame, and tempeh — these foods can vary in carbohydrates substantially, so read labels carefully; soybeans are fewer in carbs than most other beans, with only about 1–3 net carb grams per 1/2 cup serving cooked

Nuts and Seeds

- Macadamia nuts, pecans, walnuts, hazelnuts, cashews, pine nuts, sunflower seeds, pistachios, chestnuts, pumpkin seeds — 1.5–4 grams net carbs per 1 ounce; cashews are the highest in carbs, around 7 net grams per ounce
- Nut butters and seed butters — 4 net carbs per 2 tablespoons
- Chia seeds and flaxseeds — around 1–2 grams net carbs per 2 tablespoons

Fruits

Although it's widely noted that keto and fruit don't mix, because the sweet fructose in fruit is still a sugar, the fruits noted below are low in sugar and have a low impact on blood glucose and insulin responses. Eat in moderation/small quantities!

- Berries, including blueberries, strawberries, blackberries, raspberries — 3–9 grams net carbs per 1/2 cup
- Asian pears — 8–9 net carbs per pear

- Kiwis — 7.9 net carbs per kiwi
- Lemons
- Limes

Keto Snacks

Sometimes, you just need a little something to get you by. In general, we do not recommend snacking, because many people mindlessly eat when they snack and end up consuming more than intended or more than they realize as they absentmindedly keep putting food in their mouth. That said, if you need some calories and don't want or need a full meal, thoughtfully having some of the following snacks should satiate your hunger but help keep you in ketosis!

- Protein smoothie (protein powder blended with unsweetened almond milk or water)
- Berries and heavy whipping cream (no sugar added)
- Dark chocolate (at least 80% cacao)
- 7–10 olives
- Pickles
- Veggie sticks and cream cheese
- 1 tablespoon nut butter or handful of nuts
- Veggies with melted cheese
- Coconut chips
- Avocado
- Cold cuts
- Nuts
- Eggs
- Cheese
- All types of jerky (read labels; many commercial jerky products have added sugar as a flavoring)
- Pork rinds

Condiments

Most condiments listed below range from 0.5–2 net carb grams per 1–2 tablespoon serving. Check ingredient labels to make sure added sugar is not included, which will increase net carbs. (Stevia and erythritol will become your go-to sweeteners because neither raise your blood sugar — combine for a more natural sweet taste and, remember, a little goes a long way!)

Section VI

- Low carb ketchup or salsa (no sugar added)
- Sour cream
- Mustard, hot sauces, Worcestershire sauce
- Lemon/ lime juice
- Soy sauce
- Salad dressing (ideal to make your own with vinegar, oil and spices)
- Pickles – opt for cultured (made with salt not vinegar)

Sweeteners

Sugar Alcohols:
Sugar alcohols are non-calorie, low- or no-carb sweeteners that are not absorbed by the body – that's why they have little or no carb impact. So you'll see a lot of keto recipes with these sorts of sweeteners listed. The following sugar alcohols do not count toward net carbs and therefore, you don't need to count them in your daily total carb count:

- Erythritol
- Xylitol
- Mannitol
- Lactitol

Other keto-acceptable sweeteners include:

- Stevia
- Monk Fruit sweetener

We do not suggest artificial sweeteners such as aspartame, sucralose, and saccharin (most commercial no calorie sweeteners) because there has been a lot of controversy that these kinds of sweeteners not only have potential negative health effects, but in some cases, they can trick your body into thinking it's getting sugar and it releases insulin just like it does with sugar. Studies have been conflicting and controversial. Saccharin was originally found to be linked to bladder cancer in animal studies, but was eventually cleared of any such link in humans. Still, we prefer to focus on the list above. Interestingly, we've found that the longer we adhere to a low-carb, low-sugar way of eating, the more our "sweet tooth" cravings seem to go away!

Drinks

Consume the unsweetened drinks below only moderately. These will typically contain between 1–7 net carb grams per serving.

- Fresh vegetable juice
- Unsweetened coconut or almond milk (ideal to make your own)
- Bone broth, regular broth (this is helpful with electrolyte maintenance)

Miscellaneous Foods That Are Keto Friendly

- Olives
- Pickles (unsweetened)
- Cocoa powder (unsweetened)
- Dark chocolate (80% or more cacao)
- Shiratake noodles (zero carb noodles)
- Kelp noodles (zero carb noodles)
- Keto friendly protein bars (read labels; avoid sugar and carbs and only eat bars made with whole intact food ingredients)

Foods To Avoid And/Or Limit On The Ketogenic Diet

Any Type of Sugar

This may seem obvious after all our rants about sugar, but the fact is, sugar is added to so many packaged foods, and a little goes a long way! One teaspoon of sugar has about 4 grams of carbs, while every tablespoon has about 12 grams. Many products try to tout natural sugars such as "cane syrup" or "agave nectar" but sugar is sugar, no matter how natural the source. Here are examples of common sugars and their many names:

- White, brown, cane, raw and confectioner's sugar.
- Syrups like maple, carob, corn, caramel and fruit
- Honey and agave
- Any food made with ingredients ending in 'ose' such as fructose,

glucose, maltose, dextrose and lactose

Any and All Grains

One slice of bread, or small serving of grains, can have anywhere from 10–30 net grams of carbs! Cereals and cooked grains typically have 15–35 grams per 1/4 cup uncooked, depending on the kind. These foods have no place in a healthy keto lifestyle!

- Wheat, oats, all rice (white, brown, jasmine), quinoa, couscous, pilaf, etc.
- Corn and all products containing corn, including popcorn, tortillas, grits, polenta, corn flour and corn meal
- All types of products made with flour, including bread, bagels, rolls, muffins, pasta, wraps, etc.

Most Non-Berry Fruits

Most fruits simply contain too many carbs and can prevent you from reaching your goals if you eat them. So when on keto, stay away from the "sweet fruits" like mangoes, papayas, watermelon, bananas, oranges and red or yellow apples (green apples have a little less sugar in them, but still pack a decent carb punch, so eat in small quantities). Many people worry that they won't get enough vitamin C, fiber, or other micronutrients, but if you are eating veggies, you'll get all the vitamins and fiber you need, without the sugar of fruit.

Nearly All Processed Foods

- Crackers, chips, pretzels, etc.
- All types of candy
- All desserts like cookies, cakes, pies, ice cream
- Pancakes, waffles and other baked breakfast items
- Oatmeal and cereals
- Snack carbs, granola bars, most protein bars or meal replacements, etc.
- Canned soups, boxed foods, any prepackaged meal
- Foods containing artificial ingredients like artificial sweeteners (sucralose, aspartame, etc.), dyes and flavors

Sweetened and Caloric Beverages

- Soda
- Alcohol (especially beer, sweet wine, and flavored spirits or mixed drinks with sugary mixers). Occasional consumption of some types is ok (see the chapter "What About Booze" for more info!).
- Sweetened teas or coffee drinks
- Fruit juices

Although this is not an exhaustive list, we hope it helps lay the groundwork for you to start eating in a keto-friendly manner compatible with the Ketogenic Key lifestyle!

Also, this book provides some recipes to give you an idea of what sorts of meals you can eat and still maintain ketosis. We also recommend you check out some of the excellent keto cookbooks available online and at bookstores. For example, the recipe books by keto expert Maria Emmerich are creative, keto-friendly, and absolutely delicious!!

Chapter 23. What About Booze? Alcohol and Keto

Some of the most common questions we get when people ask about ketogenic therapies and the ketogenic diet are along the lines of, "What about booze? Will I have to stop drinking to get into or stay in ketosis? And, if so, for how long? Can I cheat on the weekends? Are there keto-friendly alcoholic drinks?" These are great questions, and ones that underscore the balance one needs to have between the discipline required to get healthier, and being able to indulge in things you enjoy in life. So the answer is a very definite, yes and no. Well, maybe! Let's talk about it.

The bottom line is that some alcohol consumption is possible for folks trying to achieve and stay in a state of ketosis. But you have to be careful about what and how much you drink – not all alcohol is created equal by keto standards! It also depends on what your goals are. If you're trying to lose fat, then we recommend you avoid alcohol as much as possible, at least until you hit your goal. But that doesn't mean you have to live like a monk.

In 2014, author Steve Welch did a low-carb (he wasn't fully into keto yet) body transformation program where he cut carbs and lost about 35 pounds in 16 weeks, in order to achieve the goal of having a nice 6-pack of abs by his 50th birthday. He approached alcohol this way as he wrote in a blog post at the time:

> *"I limited my alcohol consumption to once a week, and even then, I planned it as part of my weekly cheat meal. There really isn't a place for frequent boozing in your nutrition plan if you're trying to maximize your fat loss. But let's be honest, a little bit isn't going to kill you or derail your whole program.*
>
> *Prior to doing the GetFitLean program, I drank multiple times a week – usually food-oriented drinking (a couple beers at a burger joint, a nice red wine with a grilled steak, a margarita or two with some Mexican food, and so on). And you know*

what? Alcohol has calories. And that frequent alcohol consumption definitely contributed to my slow and steady weight gain that had me close to 190 pounds and sporting a gut at the age of 49."

It's an excellent point: if you're trying to get really fit and lean, alcoholic beverages aren't going to mesh into your lifestyle very well for a variety of reasons that we'll get to shortly. On the other hand, we live in a socially oriented, alcohol-friendly society, and unless you're in serious training for an athletic event, most people are not going to stop drinking completely. Steve's own personal goal was to get into great shape for his 50th birthday and beyond, not to live like a monk and forsake everything he enjoyed – and he succeeded in getting his 6-pack of abs on his 50th birthday, which simply proves that it's possible to find that balance.

But that begged a couple questions – how much is too much? Is any amount of alcohol "OK" for the purposes of the Ketogenic Key program?

The Effects of Alcohol on Fitness and Fat Loss

There's an excellent article on the hardcore bodybuilding site T-Nation called "The Lifter's Guide to Alcohol" that reviews the science around how alcohol impacts a number of health and fitness aspects, from muscle performance, fat burning, and the effects on hormone levels and the endocrine system. But here are a few of the key points that are relevant for fat loss and general fitness, since most people reading this book are probably not competitive weight lifters or bodybuilders.

Alcohol Consumption and Fat Loss

A number of factors can make this a little confusing and controversial. Some studies indicate that when you consume alcohol and have food in your system (from an earlier meal or from eating and drinking together), your body will burn alcohol calories first. Your body doesn't store alcohol or the by-products of alcohol as fat, even though many people think it does. But what that means for fat loss is, your body isn't burning the *other* calories you're consuming and *those* calories may be more likely to be stored as fat.

Therefore, alcohol may be more accurately classified as a suppressor of fat loss rather than a substance that will be stored as fat when you consume it, and may cause you to retain fat rather than burn it.

Research also suggests that the effects of alcohol on fat retention also depend on what kind of alcohol or cocktail you're drinking. Not all alcoholic drinks are created equal from a keto standpoint. A sugary and carb calorie-laden margarita is setting you up for that blood sugar spike, insulin response, and subsequent fat storage. As a result, those calories from the drink(s), in addition to calories of any food you might be consuming, will likely end up on your waistline and thighs. The T-Nation article referenced above recommends that you consume primarily protein when you're drinking alcohol and avoid carbs and fats, so that you minimize the likelihood of those calories being stored as body fat.

Alcohol Glycemic Impact

The other thing to consider when drinking is the glycemic impact of the type of alcohol you're consuming. Glycemic impact means how much it spikes your blood sugar (blood glucose), which can set you up for fat storage. The lower the glycemic impact, the better.

Spirits: Clear pure spirits like vodka and gin have no carbs, so no glycemic impact. Brown spirits (whiskey, bourbon, rye, scotch) are also low glycemically. Of course, that's if you drink them straight (neat) or on the rocks. What you mix with the booze has a big impact as well. Tonic contains sugar, where as soda water does not. So some keto proponents say it's ok to have a vodka soda or two. Just don't mix spirits with sugar and carb-laden orange juice or other sweet sugary mixers.

Wine: Dry red and white wines are typically low carb and have a minimal glycemic impact. Sweet white wines and dessert wines are typically not keto-friendly. You're probably ok having a glass or two of dry wine, but you may want to experiment with different brands and varietals. Many winemakers now tweak their wines to be a little sweeter, to counter the higher alcohol content typical of today's wines.

Beer: Beer is pretty much liquid bread, and even some light beers have a fair amount of carbs. We recommend avoiding beer if you're trying to keep your carbs low.

The Effects of Alcohol on Willpower

A potential problem with alcohol is it can impact your mental and emotional inhibition system, meaning that when you're under the influence of alcohol, you may be more likely to have cravings and eat junk that you wouldn't normally eat – this is a real concern when you're on a program like The Ketogenic Key and trying to eat effectively and smartly. Some legitimate studies have shown that drinking alcohol resulted in increased cravings for carbohydrates and sugar (no wonder that chocolate cake for dessert seems like such a "good idea" after you've had a few drinks!). So be cognizant of the potential effects of consuming alcohol, and plan your moderate alcohol consumption just like you would any other part of your nutrition. Again, our recommendation is to incorporate it into a cheat meal, and if you are tracking macros and calories, you should log any booze consumption into your MyFitnessPal or other macro tracker just like you would any other food. Be honest and transparent about what you're consuming.

Hormonal Impact: Is Booze a Testosterone Killer?

It's been broadly noted that alcohol can impact testosterone levels in a negative way, and testosterone (which is present in men and women) is a key hormone for building and maintaining lean muscle. So it makes sense that you'd want to minimize your alcohol consumption just for that reason alone. However, there's some controversy as to how much alcohol it takes to make a meaningful impact – some studies even showed that moderate drinking after weight lifting actually resulted in *increased* testosterone levels. But individuals differ in how their bodies react to things and there are numerous factors that can impact hormone levels, including stress and environmental factors. Alcohol has also been shown to lower human growth hormone (HGH) levels in the body (another naturally secreted hormone that helps you build muscle and burn fat), so that's another argument for minimizing your intake. It's also important to note that alcohol will rob your body of B-vitamins and other key nutrients, so be sure you're taking a good vitamin supplement if you drink. In the end, the jury is still out on the testosterone issue, but it's best to practice moderation and be conservative in your drinking.

A Word of Caution

One thing that is being increasingly reported is that when you're doing keto, alcohol has a much stronger impact on you because its absorption into your blood stream isn't hampered by heavy carb-laden meals. So people have reported that they get buzzed or drunk (and impaired) with half the alcohol they would normally consume. So be careful, be aware of how much alcohol you are consuming, and never drive when drinking. There have been some anecdotal reports of people on keto blowing "high" on a blood-alcohol-content (BAC) meter. Perhaps this is because ketones metabolize to the breath, especially acetone, and could be read as alcohol by some types of BAC meters (note that many BAC meters claim that they do not detect acetone as alcohol). Although somewhat controversial, this is still something to be aware of if you are doing keto and plan to drink alcohol.

Summary

The bottom line is that we strongly recommend keeping your alcohol intake as low as possible, especially if your goal is fat loss and you're trying to build a strong foundational base of healthy habits. But we also know that there are times when you want to indulge. Again, the key is finding balance. Don't use this as an excuse to slam a dozen Jaeger bombs every Saturday night or pound down a 12-pack of suds as part of a "cheat meal," making your ability to get up and exercise the next day highly unlikely. Be smart, enjoy an occasional low-carb drink or two when appropriate, and stick with the Ketogenic Key program. If you're diligent about your keto nutrition and are getting your activity in, you will make the progress you desire!

Chapter 24. Fiber and Quality Sources

Many people are familiar with the word fiber and may know it as "roughage" or "bulk." When Grandma said to eat your roughage, she was right! We know that we need fiber, two types: soluble and insoluble fiber, so the natural concern that you may be lacking fiber when reducing your food intake or carbohydrate load may arise. There is also pre-biotic fiber, which contributes to a healthy gut biome, so you may want to include that in your nutrition plan as well.

Fiber has a host of benefits including:
- Improving Gut Health
- Improving Digestion
- Heart Health
- Blood Sugar Regulation
- Possible Cancer Prevention
- Longevity

Many people, before starting the Ketogenic Key, relied upon carbohydrates such as grains or fruit for their fiber needs. Which is why one of the main questions we get when people want to start the Ketogenic Key lifestyle is, "What about fiber? Where do I get it? How can I eat fiber and maintain ketosis?"

First and very importantly, fiber in and of itself will not take you out of ketosis. Dietary fiber is a kind of carbohydrate, but it resists digestion and absorption and may or may not undergo microbial fermentation in the large intestine. Let's go over the different kinds of fiber, and some common sources of them that would be keto-friendly.

Soluble Fiber

The biggest difference between the two main types of fiber (soluble fiber and insoluble fiber) is that soluble fiber dissolves in water and very importantly, in your gut. This type of fiber, once it reaches your gut, dissolves into a gel-like substance that puts the brakes on appetite, keeping your blood sugar and insulin from spiking after we eat. The blood sugar and insulin spike is called the "postprandial spike," and we want to do our best to minimize it, as it is an important component to body weight control, and repeated spikes are believed to contribute to the development of oxidative stress and inflammation, diabetes, and cardiovascular disease. Since they help control this spike, it's not surprising that both soluble and insoluble fiber decrease inflammation.

Quality Sources of Soluble Fiber

Almonds
Avocados
Berries
Broccoli
Cabbage
Kale
Zucchini
Squash
Carrots
Sweet Potatoes
Glucomannan (fiber powder from the root of the konjac plant)

(NOTE: berries, root vegetables, carrots, and sweet potatoes can be high in carbs if eaten in significant quantities, so we suggest you go sparingly on these or get your fiber from a source that's lower in carbs).

Insoluble Fiber

Insoluble fiber is exactly what it sounds like – it does not dissolve in the intestines, and is thought to be an excellent fiber to tamp down on the hunger hormone ghrelin, due to its insoluble bulk acting as an appetite suppressant. It also has more of an anti-inflammatory effect than soluble fiber.

Additionally, insoluble fiber speeds up the passage of food through the digestive system. This helps maintain regularity and prevent constipation.

Research shows that insoluble fiber may directly promote fat loss. One study (done on mice) showed that the mice fed a soluble fiber diet became obese and pre-diabetic. Yet, when the researchers used insoluble fiber, the mice did not gain as much weight due to better fat metabolism. The bottom line is that insoluble fiber may help you lose weight and prevent weight gain. If weight loss is part of your personal Ketogenic Key goals, load up on insoluble fiber.

Quality Sources of Insoluble Fiber:

Kale
Collard Greens
Green Beans
Celery
Leeks
Green Onions
Cabbage
Broccoli
Cauliflower
Brussels Sprouts
Almonds
Walnuts

Prebiotic Fiber

Prebiotic fiber is a key player in optimizing gut health. This special fiber ferments in your gut feeding your healthy gut bugs instead of just passing through relatively intact as other fiber types mainly do. We like to refer to prebiotic fiber as fertilizer for your healthy gut garden. When the microflora are fed well, they break down the fiber into short-chain fatty acids that fight inflammation and promote the integrity of the gut lining. Research shows prebiotic fiber has a host of health benefits that includes weight loss due to a healthy microbiome.

Quality Sources of Prebiotic Fiber

Raw Dandelion Greens
Raw Garlic
Leeks
Jerusalem Artichokes
Raw Jicama
Chicory Root

Chapter 24. Fiber and Quality Sources

Emerging (and controversial?) Hypothesis About Fiber

There is an interesting movement right now that claims fiber is in fact not necessary for optimal health. The proponents of this hypothesis suggest that while fiber may be doing all sorts of good things for our body, heart, and gut healthy, it's because we've been eating all the wrong things for so long – so it's almost like fiber is being used to help undo the damage we've done. They suggest that if you follow a low-carb, low-sugar, high-fat ketogenic diet, your body won't need fiber, and it becomes an unnecessary nutrient to try to work into your nutritional plans. This is an interesting train of thinking that may have merit, and bears watching. As more people adopt keto, we will likely find out more and more about what is and is not necessary nutritionally.

We've also had people ask us, what if you choose to eat an all-meat, zero-carb diet such as the Carnivore Diet? It is important to note that fiber isn't the only source of short-chain fatty acids so necessary to for optimal health. We can, and do, make them out of proteins as well. Short-chain fatty acids are the main source of nutrition for the microflora in your colon. SCFAs may reduce the risk of inflammatory diseases, type 2 diabetes, obesity, heart disease and other conditions.

Summary

It is our opinion that fiber can be an important part of a healthy lifestyle, especially if you need to balance or improve gut health and colon health. It will be interesting to watch this topic evolve as more studies are done on low carb, ketogenic, and whole food diets to see whether fiber is truly necessary as we've been led to believe, or is it only necessary because we've been eating so much carbohydrate laden, highly processed foods for the past century?

Section VI. Part II: Recipes

The recipes we've included in the following chapters are simple, and are really just basic guides. Ultimately, you should experiment and modify them to your tastes. In addition, some things in these recipes may not agree with you. For example, we know some people are very sensitive to erythritol zero calorie sweeteners and get GI upset from them. If that's the case, feel free to substitute stevia powder or drops, to your level of sweetness. Ditto for any other ingredients that may not agree with you. Also, none of these recipes include much spice, so by all means feel free to jazz some of them up with salsa, Cholula or Tabasco sauce, red pepper flakes, or any other flavorful spice that you think will make a recipe mouth-watering for you. Food should be delicious and fun to make! Ready? Let's dig in!

Chapter 25. Breakfast Recipes

KETO BREAKFAST MUFFINS

Serves: *6-8*
Prep Time: *10*   Minutes
Cook Time: *15*   Minutes
Total Time: *25*   Minutes

INGREDIENTS

- 1 cup almond flour
- 1 large egg
- ¼ cup vanilla almond milk

- 2 tablespoons erythritol sweetener or use some stevia drops (to your taste)
- 1 tsp vanilla extract
- ½ tablespoon baking powder

DIRECTIONS

1. Preheat oven to 325 F
2. In a bowl blend all ingredients and mix well
3. Add the rest of ingredients and mix
4. Pour batter into well-oiled 6-8 cupcake tin and bake for 15-18 minutes
5. Remove and serve

KETO PANCAKES

Serves: *4*

Prep Time:	*10*	Minutes
Cook Time:	*10*	Minutes
Total Time:	*20*	Minutes

INGREDIENTS

- ½ cup almond flour
- 3 eggs
- ½ tsp cinnamon
- 1 tablespoon butter
- ½ cup cream cheese

DIRECTIONS

1. Place all ingredients in a bowl and mix using a blender
2. In a frying pan pour 2-3 tablespoons of pancake mixture and cook for 1-2 minutes per side
3. Remove and top with cinnamon or butter

Chapter 25. Breakfast Recipes

BREAKFAST SANDWICH

Serves: *1*
Prep Time: **5**   Minutes
Cook Time: **5**   Minutes
Total Time: **10**   Minutes

INGREDIENTS

- 3 tablespoons shredded cheddar cheese
- 1 egg
- 1 slice bacon
- Salt and pepper to taste

DIRECTIONS

1. In a skillet add shredded cheese oven medium heat and remove to a paper towel when it starts to melt (it will form a thin cheese "shell" as it cools)
2. Cook the egg as you want
3. Remove cooked egg and place it over a section of the cheese shell and season with salt and pepper
4. Place the remaining cheese shell over the top and serve

POWER BREAKFAST RINGS WITH GREEN SAUCE

Serves: *3*
Prep Time: *10*   Minutes
Cook Time: *10*   Minutes
Total Time: *20*   Minutes

INGREDIENTS

- **1 cup baby spinach**
- **Salt to taste**
- **1 cup parsley**
- **4 garlic cloves**
- **4 tablespoons hemp hearts**
- **1 cup olive oil**
- **-4 slices bacon**
- **1 cup arugula**
- **1 egg**
- **-10 asparagus tips**

DIRECTIONS

1. **For green sauce, mix arugula, olive oil, parsley, garlic cloves, baby spinach, hemp hearts in a blender and blend until smooth**
2. **Arrange bacon sliced into rings and place the bacon in the oven at 325 F and cook until done**
3. **Tuck 3-4 asparagus tips into each bacon ring and add green sauce, sprinkle salt and pepper and cook for another 12-15 minutes**
4. **Remove from oven and serve**

Chapter 25. Breakfast Recipes

PEPPER RINGS

Serves: *2*
Prep Time: **10** Minutes
Cook Time: **10** Minutes
Total Time: **20** Minutes

INGREDIENTS

- **2 red bell peppers**
- **Salt (to taste)**
- **Pepper (to taste)**
- **6 eggs**
- **1 lb breakfast sausage**
- **3 tablespoons parmesan cheese**

DIRECTIONS

1. **In a skillet, brown breakfast sausage and set aside**
2. **Cut peppers into 6 rings and place them in the skillet and cook**
3. **Pour an egg into each ring and add salt and sausage inside the yolk of each ring**
4. **Sprinkle with parmesan cheese**
5. **When ready remove and serve**

KETO EGG BITES

Serves: **2**
Prep Time: **10**   Minutes
Cook Time: **20**   Minutes
Total Time: **30**   Minutes

INGREDIENTS

- **4 eggs**
- **½ cup shredded Swiss cheese**
- **½ cup full-fat cottage cheese**
- **½ tsp salt**
- **Black pepper**
- **2 thick slices of paleo sugar-free bacon**

DIRECTIONS

1. **Preheat oven to 325 F**
2. **In a bowl mix cottage cheese, salt, pepper, cheese, eggs and blend until smooth**
3. **Spray a muffin tin and pour the mixture into it, add chopped bacon and bake for 25 minutes**
4. **Remove and serve**

Chapter 25. Breakfast Recipes

BREAKFAST BOWL

Serves: *1*
Prep Time: *10*   Minutes
Cook Time: *10*   Minutes
Total Time: *20*   Minutes

INGREDIENTS

- **2 eggs**
- **2 strips bacon, chopped**
- **½ cup shredded cheddar cheese**
- **½ cup salsa**
- **2 tablespoons butter**
- **½ avocado, sliced**

DIRECTIONS

1. **In a bowl scramble the eggs and place them into the skillet, cook for 2-3 minutes**
2. **Top the eggs with shredded cheese and chopped bacon**
3. **Slice avocado and place it over the bacon**
4. **Top with salsa and serve**

   Tip: if you like Cholula sauce, use it instead of salsa

KETO BREAKFAST "POTATOES"

Serves: **4**
Prep Time: **10**   Minutes
Cook Time: **10**   Minutes
Total Time: **20**   Minutes

INGREDIENTS

* 1 large turnip
* ½ tsp paprika, garlic powder, salt
* 1 tsp parsley
* ½ cup onion, chopped
* 2 slices bacon, chopped
* 1 tablespoon olive oil

DIRECTIONS

1. In a skillet add the turnips and spices, cook for 5-6 minutes, add onion and cook for another 2-3 minutes
2. Chop the bacon and add to the skillet, cook for another 2-3 minutes
3. Remove to a place and top with parsley before serving

Chapter 25. Breakfast Recipes

MINI BREAKFAST MEATLOAFS

Serves: *4*
Prep Time: *10*   Minutes
Cook Time: *30*   Minutes
Total Time: *40*   Minutes

INGREDIENTS

- 1 lb pork sausage
- 1 egg
- 1 cup shredded cheddar cheese
- 4 slices bacon, chopped
- 4 slices ham, diced

DIRECTIONS

1. Preheat oven to 325 F
2. In a bowl mix all ingredients
3. Divide mixture into 6-8 portions and pack into mini loaf pan cavities
4. Bake for 30 minutes, remove and serve

KETO JALAPENO MUFFINS

Serves: *4*
Prep Time: *10*   Minutes
Cook Time: *30*   Minutes
Total Time: *40*   Minutes

INGREDIENTS

- **8 eggs**
- **8 oz cheddar cheese**
- **¾ cup heavy cream**
- **1 tsp salt**
- **1 tsp jalapeno, chopped**
- **8 slices bacon**

DIRECTIONS

1. **Preheat oven to 325**
2. **Add one slice of bacon to bottom of each muffin tin**
3. **In a bowl mix cream, cheese, pepper, eggs and salt**
4. **Distribute into 8-10 muffin cups and add jalapeno to each muffin tin**
5. **Bake for 15-20 minutes, when ready remove and serve**

Chapter 26. Lunch Recipes

SOUP RECIPES

KETO BROCCOLI SOUP

Serves: *4*
Prep Time: *10*   Minutes
Cook Time: *30*   Minutes
Total Time: *40*   Minutes

INGREDIENTS

- 2 tablespoons olive oil
- 1 cup chicken broth
- 1 cup heavy whipping cream
- 6 oz shredded cheddar cheese
- 1 tsp salt
- 5 oz broccoli, chopped
- 1 celery stalk, diced
- 1 small carrot, diced
- ½ onion, chopped

DIRECTIONS

1. In a pot add olive oil over medium heat
2. Add onion, carrot, celery and cook for 2-3 minutes
3. Add chicken broth and simmer for 4-5 minutes
4. Stir in broccoli and cream
5. Sprinkle in cheese and season with salt

KETO TACO SOUP

Serves: **8**
Prep Time: **10**   Minutes
Cook Time: **10**   Minutes
Total Time: **20**   Minutes

INGREDIENTS

- 2 lbs ground beef
- 1 onion, diced
- 1 cup heavy whipping cream
- 1 tsp chili powder
- 14 oz. cream cheese
- 1 tsp garlic
- 1 tsp cumin
- 2 ten oz. canned tomatoes, chopped
- 16 oz. beef broth

DIRECTIONS

1. Cook beef until browned, add in onion, garlic and simmer until softened
2. Add cream cheese and stir until fully melted
3. Add tomatoes, whipping cream, beef broth, stir and bring to boil then simmer for 20 minutes.

Chapter 26. Lunch Recipes

SLOW COOKER KETO CHICKEN SOUP

Serves: **4**
Prep Time: **10** Minutes
Cook Time: **30** Minutes
Total Time: **40** Minutes

INGREDIENTS

- 2 boneless chicken breasts
- 20-ounces canned tomatoes, diced
- ½ tsp salt
- 1 cup salsa
- 6-ounces cream cheese, diced
- 1 avocado, diced
- 2 tablespoons taco seasoning
- 1.5 cups chicken broth

DIRECTIONS

1. In a slow cooker place all ingredients and cook for 5-6 hours or until chicken is tender
2. Whisk cream cheese into the broth
3. When ready, remove and serve

KETO SPINACH SOUP

Serves: *2*
Prep Time: *5*   Minutes
Cook Time: *15*   Minutes
Total Time: *20*   Minutes

INGREDIENTS

- ¼ lbs spinach
- 2 oz onion, chopped
- ¼ cup heavy cream
- ½ oz garlic
- 1 chicken stock cube
- 1.5 cups chicken broth
- 1 tablespoons butter

DIRECTIONS

1. In a saucepan melt the butter and sauté the onion
2. Add garlic, spinach and stock cube and half the broth
3. Cook until spinach wilts
4. Pour everything in a blender and blend (or use an immersion blender), add rest of broth
5. Serve with pepper and toasted nuts of choice

Chapter 26. Lunch Recipes

KETO TOSCANA SOUP

Serves: *4*
Prep Time: *10*   Minutes
Cook Time: *30*   Minutes
Total Time: *40*   Minutes

INGREDIENTS
* **1 lb Italian sausage**
* **2 tablespoons olive oil**
* **½ cup heavy whipping cream**
* **1 tsp garlic**
* **2 cup kale leaves, chopped**
* **1 16 oz bag radishes, sliced**
* **1 onion, chopped**
* **4 cups vegetable broth**

DIRECTIONS

1. **Slice radishes and blend until smooth**
2. **In a hot pot add olive oil, onion and sausage, cook until sausage is browned, and onions have softened, add radishes and broth**
3. **Cook on medium heat, add heavy whipping cream, kale leaves**
4. **Simmer on stove for 20 minutes**
5. **Remove and serve**

KETO PARMESAN SOUP

Serves: *4*
Prep Time: *10*   Minutes
Cook Time: *30*   Minutes
Total Time: *40*   Minutes

INGREDIENTS

- 1 lb broccoli, chopped
- 1 tablespoon butter
- 1 tablespoon parmesan cheese
- 1 onion, chopped
- 4 cups chicken broth
- 1 tsp salt
- 1 tsp pepper
- ½ cup heavy cream

DIRECTIONS

1. In a saucepan add onion and sauté until softened
2. Stir in broccoli and cook until soft
3. Combine with heavy cream and place in a blender, blend until smooth
4. Return to the saucepan, add chicken broth
5. Stir and simmer for 20 minutes
6. Season with salt and pepper
7. Sprinkle with parmesan and serve

Chapter 26. Lunch Recipes

KETO CAULIFLOWER SOUP

Serves: *4*
Prep Time: *10*   Minutes
Cook Time: *30*   Minutes
Total Time: *40*   Minutes

INGREDIENTS

- ½ head of cauliflower, chopped
- 1 tablespoon butter
- ½ cup heavy cream
- ½ red bell pepper, finely diced
- 1 tsp salt
- 1 tsp pepper
- 1 tablespoons parmesan cheese
- 4 cups chicken broth
- 1 tsp Italian herbs

DIRECTIONS

1. In a large saucepan melt butter, add cauliflower and cook until soft
2. Remove from saucepan and set aside
3. Melt butter and sauté bell pepper
4. In a food processor add cauliflower mixture, red pepper
5. Season with salt and pepper
6. Add vegetables and chicken broth
7. Simmer for 20 minutes
8. Garnish with parmesan and serve

KETO BROCCOLI CHEESE SOUP

Serves: *2*
Prep Time: *10*   Minutes
Cook Time: *20*   Minutes
Total Time: *30*   Minutes

INGREDIENTS

- 2 cups broccoli, chopped
- 3 cups chicken broth
- 1 onion, chopped
- 1 cup heavy cream
- 6 oz cream cheese
- 1 tablespoon hot sauce
- 3 tablespoons butter
- 1 clove garlic, minced
- 6 oz cheddar cheese, diced

DIRECTIONS

1. In a saucepan melt butter, add onion, garlic and sauté until soft
2. Pour in heavy cream, chicken broth, stir in broccoli
3. Cover, bring to a simmer and continue cooking for 12-15 minutes
4. Add cheese, stir and cook until melted,
5. Stir in hot sauce and enjoy

Chapter 26. Lunch Recipes

KETO CHICKEN QUESO SOUP

Serves: **4**
Prep Time: **10** Minutes
Cook Time: **30** Minutes
Total Time: **40** Minutes

INGREDIENTS

- -1 lb chicken breast or dark thigh meat, cubed
- 1 tablespoon taco seasoning
- 1 tablespoon avocado oil
- 1 can diced green chilies
- 6-ounces cream cheese
- ½ cup heavy cream
- 1 tsp salt
- 1 tsp pepper
- 4 cups chicken broth
- ½ cup shredded cheddar

DIRECTIONS

1. In a Dutch oven heat oil over medium heat.
2. Stir in taco seasoning and cook for 1-2 minutes
3. Add broth, chicken and simmer for 20 minutes, remove chicken and shred
4. Stir in cream cheese and heavy cream into the soup, once the cheese has melted, add the chicken back to the soup, sprinkle shredded cheddar on top, season with salt and freshly ground pepper. Serve.

KETO CRAB SOUP

Serves: **6**
Prep Time: **10**   Minutes
Cook Time: **10**   Minutes
Total Time: **20**   Minutes

INGREDIENTS

- **1 tablespoon butter**
- **1 tablespoon seafood seasoning**
- **½ tsp salt**
- **½ tsp pepper**
- **6 oz cream cheese**
- **¾ cup parmesan cheese**
- **1 lb lump crabmeat**
- **4 cups chicken broth**

DIRECTIONS

1. **In a pot melt butter and add seafood seasoning, salt and pepper, cream cheese and whisk until smooth**
2. **Add chicken broth and bring to a boil**
3. **Add parmesan cheese, crab meat and reduce heat**
4. **Simmer 20 minutes.**
5. **Remove and serve**

Chapter 27. Salad Recipes

KETO CHICKEN AND BACON SALAD

Serves: *2*
Prep Time: *10*   Minutes
Cook Time: *10*   Minutes
Total Time: *20*   Minutes

INGREDIENTS

- 1 slice pan-fried bacon, chopped
- 3 oz cooked chicken breast or thigh, diced
- ½ cup shredded cheddar cheese
- 2 tablespoons olive oil
- 1 tablespoon apple cider vinegar
- ½ avocado, diced
- 1 head romaine lettuce, chopped or torn
- Salt and pepper to taste

DIRECTIONS

1. Chop all ingredients and place them in a bowl
2. Mix well and add pepper, oil and vinegar

Note: Cooked Chicken Breast can be plain, or seasoned to your liking. Blackened, Jerk, or Buffalo!

KETO BROCCOLI SALAD

Serves: *2*
Prep Time: *10*   Minutes
Cook Time: *10*   Minutes
Total Time: *20*   Minutes

INGREDIENTS

- 20 oz raw broccoli heads, chopped if large
- 1 cup pan-fried bacon, chopped
- ½ red onion, chopped
- 1 cup avocado mayo
- 1 cup macadamia nuts
- ½ tsp monk fruit sweetener
- 1 tablespoon organic apple cider vinegar

DIRECTIONS

1. Place macadamia nuts in a blender and blend until smooth
2. Place all ingredients in a bowl and mix well, pour macadamia nuts mixture over salad mixture and serve

Chapter 27. Salad Recipes

KETO GREEN SPRING SALAD

Serves: **4**
Prep Time: **10**   Minutes
Cook Time: **30**   Minutes
Total Time: **40**   Minutes

INGREDIENTS

- **2 ounces mixed greens**
- **2 tablespoons pine nuts**
- **1 tablespoon raspberry vinaigrette**
- **1 tablespoon parmesan cheese**
- **1 slice pan-fried bacon, chopped**
- **Salt and pepper to taste**

DIRECTIONS

1. **Cook bacon until crispy. Chop.**
2. **Place greens in a bowl with the rest of ingredients and toss**
3. **Top with bacon and serve**

KETO EGG SALAD

Serves: *4*
Prep Time: *10*   Minutes
Cook Time: *30*   Minutes
Total Time: *40*   Minutes

INGREDIENTS

- 6 hard-boiled eggs, shell removed
- 2 celery stalks, finely chopped
- 2 green onion stalks, chopped
- 1 green pepper, seeded and chopped
- 1 tsp Dijon mustard
- 2/3 cup avocado mayonnaise

DIRECTIONS

1. Hard boil eggs, peel shell and place in a bowl
2. Chop green pepper, onions and celery
3. In a bowl mix all the ingredients and serve

Chapter 27. Salad Recipes

KETO CAESAR SALAD

Serves: **4**
Prep Time: **10** Minutes
Cook Time: **30** Minutes
Total Time: **40** Minutes

INGREDIENTS

- **12 oz chicken breasts, roasted and sliced**
- **1 tablespoon olive oil**
- **Salt to taste**
- **2 oz pan-fried bacon, chopped**
- **6 oz romaine lettuce, torn leaves**
- **1 oz parmesan cheese**
  DRESSING
- **½ cup mayonnaise**
- **1 tablespoon chopped anchovies**
- **1 garlic clove, finely minced**
- **1 tablespoon Dijon or yellow mustard**
- **½ lemon zest**
- **1 tablespoon parmesan cheese**

DIRECTIONS

1. **In a bowl mix all ingredients for the dressing and set aside**
2. **Preheat oven to 400 F and place chicken breast in a baking dish and bake for 15-20 minutes until browned.**
3. **In a bowl place sliced chicken, all the salad ingredients, dressing and mix well**
4. **Serve with parmesan cheese**

KETO PEPPERONI SALAD

Serves: *4*
Prep Time: *10*   Minutes
Cook Time: *30*   Minutes
Total Time: *40*   Minutes

INGREDIENTS

- ½ avocado, diced
- 12 slices pepperoni, chopped
- 1 oz mozzarella cheese, diced
- ½ tsp Italian seasoning
- Salt and pepper to taste
- 1 tablespoon olive oil

DIRECTIONS

1. In a bowl mix all ingredients and serve

Chapter 27. Salad Recipes

KETO CHICKEN SALAD

Serves: *4*
Prep Time: *10*   Minutes
Cook Time: *30*   Minutes
Total Time: *40*   Minutes

INGREDIENTS

- **2 ribs celery, chopped**
- **½ tsp pink Himalayan salt**
- **1 tsp fresh dill**
- **½ cup chopped pecans**
- **1 lb chicken breast, chopped**
- **½ cup avocado mayo**
- **1 tsp Dijon mustard**

DIRECTIONS

1. **Preheat oven to 425 F and bake chicken breast for 15-20 minutes until done.**
2. **Remove chicken and dice**
3. **In a bowl mix all ingredients and toss until chicken is fully coated**
4. **When ready, add dill and serve**

KETO TUNA SALAD

Serves: **4**
Prep Time: **10** Minutes
Cook Time: **30** Minutes
Total Time: **40** Minutes

INGREDIENTS

- 1 can tuna
- ½ tsp dill
- 1 hard-boiled egg, chopped
- 1 slice pan-fried bacon, chopped
- 1 tablespoon avocado mayo
- 1 tablespoon sour cream
- 1 tsp mustard
- 1 tablespoon onion, finely chopped

DIRECTIONS

1. Prepare bacon, onion and boil egg
2. In a bowl place tuna, add egg and onion and the rest of ingredients. Mix well.
3. Top with bacon and serve

Chapter 27. Salad Recipes

KETO SPINACH SALAD

Serves: **4**
Prep Time: **10** Minutes
Cook Time: **30** Minutes
Total Time: **20** Minutes

INGREDIENTS

- **2 cups baby spinach leaves**
- **½ avocado, diced**
- **1 strawberry, sliced**
  DRESSING

- **2 slices bacon, pan-fried and chopped**
- **1 tablespoon avocado oil**
- **Pinch red pepper flakes**
- **1 tsp oregano**
- **½ tsp garlic powder**
- **½ tsp salt**
- **Juice of one half lemon**

DIRECTIONS

1. **In a bowl mix all dressing ingredients**
2. **In another bowl mix salad ingredients and pour dressing over**
3. **Mix well and serve**

KETO "POTATO" SALAD

Serves: *1*
Prep Time: *10*   Minutes
Cook Time: *10*   Minutes
Total Time: *20*   Minutes

INGREDIENTS

- **1 small head of cauliflower florets**
- **1 tablespoon mustard**
- **1 tsp celery seeds**
- **½ tsp salt**
- **½ cup celery**
- **1 tsp dill**
- **½ cup sour cream**
- **½ cup avocado mayonnaise**
- **2 stalks green onions, chopped**
- **2 hard boiled eggs, chopped**
- **1 tablespoon white vinegar**

DIRECTIONS

1. **In a bowl prepare dressing by whisking together sour cream, celery seed, salt, mayonnaise, vinegar and mustard**
2. **In another bowl mix salad ingredients, pour dressing over and mix well**

Chapter 28. Dinner Recipes

KETO MONGOLIAN BEEF

Serves: **2**
Prep Time: **10** Minutes
Cook Time: **10** Minutes
Total Time: **20** Minutes

INGREDIENTS

- **1 lb flat iron steak, sliced**
- **½ cup coconut oil**
- **2 green onions, chopped**

LOW CARB MONGOLIAN BEEF MARINADE

- **½ cup soy sauce**
- **1 tsp freshly chopped ginger**
- **1 clove garlic, finely chopped**

DIRECTIONS

1. **Cut the flat iron steak into thin slices**
2. **Add the beef to a Ziploc bag and add soy sauce, garlic and ginger, marinate for at lease one hour**
3. **Add coconut oil to a wok or large pan and cook beef on high heat for 2-3 minutes**
4. **Add green onions, cook for another 1-2 minutes**
5. **Remove and serve**

KETO MUSHROOM PIZZA

Serves: *2*
Prep Time: **10** Minutes
Cook Time: **15** Minutes
Total Time: **25** Minutes

INGREDIENTS

* Cauliflower pizza crust, store bought
* ¼ cup store-bought marinara sauce
* 10 pepperoni slices
* 6 ounces sliced baby bella mushrooms
* 4 ounces sliced ripe olives
* ½ cup shredded mozzarella

DIRECTIONS

1. Preheat oven to 375 F
2. Spray a pie plate with a non-stick cooking spray, add pizza crust on pie plate
3. Spread marinara on top of pizza crust and mozzarella cheese
4. Layer mushrooms, pepperoni, olives and top with additional mozzarella
5. Bake for 10 minutes until cheese is melted and golden brown
6. Serve

Chapter 28. Dinner Recipes

PEPPERONI KETO PIZZA

Serves: *2*
Prep Time: **10** Minutes
Cook Time: **10** Minutes
Total Time: **20** Minutes

INGREDIENTS

- 1 cauliflower crust, store-bought
- 2 oz. pepperoni slices
- ½ cup pizza sauce or commercial marina sauce
- ½ tsp. salt
- 2-ounces fresh shredded mozzarella
- ½ cup chopped jalapenos

DIRECTIONS

1. Preheat oven to 375 F and place pizza crust on a vented pizza pan, cook for 8-10 minutes until hot
2. Add tomato sauce, pepperoni slices and jalapenos on top of the crust, sprinkle with cheese.
3. Place back in the oven for 5-6 minutes until cheese is melted, golden brown and bubbling.
4. Remove and serve

Note: We recommend baking at 375 but follow the directions on the package of your cauliflower pizza crust to ensure proper baking texture!

QUICK KETO PAN PIZZA

Serves: *4*
Prep Time: *10*   Minutes
Cook Time: *10*   Minutes
Total Time: *10*   Minutes

INGREDIENTS

PIZZA CRUST

- 2 eggs
- 1 tablespoon parmesan cheese
- 1 tablespoon psyllium husk powder
- ½ tsp Italian seasoning
- 1 tsp salt
- 2 tsp avocado oil for cooking pizza crust

TOPPINGS

- 1 oz shredded mozzarella cheese
- 2 tablespoons tomato sauce
- 1 tablespoon chopped, fresh basil

DIRECTIONS

1. In a bowl mix all pizza crust ingredients
2. Spoon the mixture into an oiled frying pan, cook about 1 minute per side or until crust texture is firm.
3. Top with cheese, tomato sauce and broil for 1-2 minutes until cheese is bubbling

BUFFALO KETO CHICKEN TENDERS

Serves: *2*
Prep Time: *10*   Minutes
Cook Time: *30*   Minutes
Total Time: *40*   Minutes

INGREDIENTS

- 1 lb chicken breast tenders cut into 1 inch pieces
- 1.5 cups finely-ground almond flour
- 1 tsp salt
- 1 tsp freshly ground pepper
- 1 tsp garlic powder
- 1 egg
- 2 tablespoons heavy whipping cream
- 5 oz buffalo sauce

DIRECTIONS

1. Preheat oven to 325 F
2. Season chicken with salt, pepper
3. Season almond flour with salt, pepper and garlic powder
4. Beat 1 egg with heavy cream
5. Dip each tender in the egg and then into seasoned almond flour
6. Place tenders on a well-oiled baking sheet. Bake for 25 minutes or until crispy
7. Remove and serve

KETO LASAGNA

Serves: *4*
Prep Time: **10**   Minutes
Cook Time: **30**   Minutes
Total Time: **40**   Minutes

INGREDIENTS

- **1 lb ground beef**
- **2 large zucchini, sliced**
- **1 cup marinara sauce**
- **¾ cup shredded mozzarella**
- **6 tablespoons ricotta cheese**
- **1 tsp salt, 1 tsp onion powder, 1 tsp Italian seasoning**

DIRECTIONS

1. **Preheat oven to 350 F, brown beef and season**
2. **Prepare zucchini noodles: Slice zucchini lengthwise into very thin slices. Sprinkle slices lightly with salt; set aside to drain in a colander.**
3. **Layer a deep dish with zucchini noodles, ricotta, marinara sauce**
4. **After layering, sprinkle with mozzarella, top with more ricotta cheese**
5. **Bake for 20-25 minutes until cheese is browned and bubbling.**
6. **Remove, serve and enjoy.**

KETO PARMESAN CHICKEN CASSEROLE

Serves: *3*
Prep Time: *10*   Minutes
Cook Time: *30*   Minutes
Total Time: *40*   Minutes

INGREDIENTS

- 2 cups cooked or rotisserie chicken, cut into 1 inch pieces
- ½ tsp dried basil
- 2 slices bacon, pan-fried and chopped
- 1 cup marinara sauce
- ½ tsp red pepper flakes
- ¾ cup shredded mozzarella cheese
- ½ cup parmesan cheese

DIRECTIONS

1. Preheat the oven to 325 F
2. Lay out the chicken in the pan and spread the marinara sauce all over
3. Top with parmesan cheese, red pepper flakes, mozzarella, chopped bacon and basil
4. Bake for 20-25 minutes, remove and serve

KETO CHEESE MEATBALLS

Serves: *2*
Prep Time: *10*   Minutes
Cook Time: *10*   Minutes
Total Time: *20*   Minutes

INGREDIENTS

- ½ lb ground beef
- 1 egg
- 2 tablespoons parmesan cheese
- ½ tsp salt
- ½ tsp pepper
- ¼ lbs cheese
- 1 tsp garlic powder

DIRECTIONS

1. Mix all ingredients with the ground beef
2. Form small meatballs
3. Add meatballs to a well-oiled pan
4. Pan fry the meatballs until done
5. Serve and enjoy

Chapter 28. Dinner Recipes

KETO CHEESY BACON CHICKEN

Serves: *4*
Prep Time: *10* Minutes
Cook Time: *30* Minutes
Total Time: *40* Minutes

INGREDIENTS

- 2 halved chicken breasts
- 2 tablespoons seasoning rub
- ½ lb bacon
- 4 oz shredded cheddar cheese
- 1 cup low-carb/no-sugar barbecue sauce

DIRECTIONS

1. Preheat oven to 375 F and spray a baking sheet with cooking spray
2. Rub both sides of chicken breast with seasoning rub, barbecue sauce and top with bacon, bake for 25 minutes
3. Remove from oven, sprinkle with cheese and serve

KETO CHEESEBURGER MEATLOAF

Serves: *2*
Prep Time: *10*   Minutes
Cook Time: *60*   Minutes
Total Time: *70*   Minutes

INGREDIENTS

- 2 lbs ground grass-fed beef
- 2 eggs
- ½ cup grated parmesan
- 1 small onion
- 1 tsp salt
- 1 tsp garlic powder
- 1 cup cheddar cheese

DIRECTIONS

1. In a bowl mix all ingredients except cheddar cheese
2. Place mixture into a sprayed oven dish and form a meatloaf shape
3. Add cheddar cheese on top of loaf
4. Bake at 325 F for 50 minutes
5. Remove and serve

Chapter 29. Dessert Recipes

CHEESECAKE KETO FAT BOMBS

Serves: *12*
Prep Time: *10*   Minutes
Cook Time: *10*   Minutes
Total Time: *20*   Minutes

INGREDIENTS

- 5 oz. cream cheese
- 2 oz. defrosted fresh strawberries (or any berries)
- 2 oz butter
- 1 oz swerve sweetener
- 1 tsp vanilla extract

DIRECTIONS

1. Puree strawberries using a blender
2. In a bowl mix Swerve sweetener, vanilla, pureed strawberries and mix well
3. Microwave cream cheese on low setting and combine with the rest of ingredients
4. Stir in melted butter (or mix with an electric mixer)
5. Divide into 10-12 round silicone molds or oiled muffin tins and freeze for 1-2 hours before serving

CHOCOLATE PEANUT BUTTER KETO FAT BOMBS

Serves: *12*
Prep Time: *10*   Minutes
Cook Time: *10*   Minutes
Total Time: *20*   Minutes

INGREDIENTS

- 4 tablespoons coconut oil
- 4 tablespoons grass-fed butter
- 4 tablespoons peanut butter (low-carb)
- 2 tablespoons unsweetened cocoa powder
- 10-12 drops of stevia liquid sweetener (or more depending on taste)
- Silicon shaped molds or ice cube molds

DIRECTIONS

1. Melt butter in microwave
2. Add coconut oil (should be liquid, warm up if necessary), peanut butter, and cocoa powder
3. Blend with immersion blender or mixer
4. Add sweetener (sweeten to taste)
5. Pour into silicone ice cube molds and freeze for 1 hour before serving (store leftover bombs in freezer; these will melt at room temperature)
6. NOTE: You can find all kinds of fun silicone ice cube molds, so get creative and have fun!

Chapter 30. Smoothie Recipes

KETO BROWNIES

Serves: **12**
Prep Time: **10** Minutes
Cook Time: **20** Minutes
Total Time: **30** Minutes

INGREDIENTS

- ½ cup finely-ground almond flour
- ½ tsp baking powder
- 1 tablespoon instant coffee
- 2 oz dark chocolate sweetened with stevia (such as Lily's brand), chopped
- 1 egg
- ½ tsp vanilla extract
- ½ cup cacao powder
- 2/3 cup erythritol sweetener
- 8 tablespoons butter

DIRECTIONS

1. Preheat oven to 325 F
2. In a medium bowl whisk almond flour, baking powder, erythritol sweetener, cocoa powder and instant coffee
3. Melt chocolate in a bowl placed over a pan of simmering water
4. Add butter and whisk in the eggs and vanilla
5. Add to dry ingredients and mix well
6. Transfer batter into baking dish and bake for 20 minutes
7. Remove and serve

KETO ICE CREAM

Serves: *2*
Prep Time: *10*   Minutes
Cook Time: *20*   Minutes
Total Time: *30*   Minutes

INGREDIENTS

- 2 cups heavy cream
- 1 tablespoon dry milk powder
- ½ tsp xanthan gum
- 1 tsp vanilla extract
- 1 cup whole milk
- ½ cup truvia baking blend sweetener

DIRECTIONS

1. In a bowl mix milk powder, sweetener, xanthan gum
2. Pour in cream, vanilla extract, milk and mix until sweetener is dissolved
3. Pour into ice cream maker and churn until set
4. Serve when ready

Chapter 30. Smoothie Recipes

KETO EGG CREPES

Serves: *2*
Prep Time: *10*   Minutes
Cook Time: *10*   Minutes
Total Time: *20*   Minutes

INGREDIENTS

- 5 eggs
- 5 oz full-fat cream cheese
- 1 tsp cinnamon
- 1 tablespoon Swerve (erythritol) sweetener
- Butter

FILLING

- 7 tablespoons butter
- ½ cup sugar substitute such as monk fruit sweetener
- 1 tablespoon cinnamon

DIRECTIONS

1. Blend all of the crepe ingredients until smooth
2. Pour batter into the pan and cook 1-2 minutes per side or until small bubbles appear.
3. For crepes topping: mix cinnamon, butter and sweetener in a bowl and spread over each crepe and roll-up.
4. Serve when ready

KETO NAAN BREAD

Serves: *4*
Prep Time: *10*   Minutes
Cook Time: *30*   Minutes
Total Time: *40*   Minutes

INGREDIENTS

- **1 cup coconut flour**
- **2 tablespoons psyllium husk**
- **2 tablespoon ghee or butter (more for pan-frying)**
- **1 tsp baking powder**
- **1 tsp salt**

DIRECTIONS

1. **In a bowl mix all ingredients**
2. **Divine the dough into 6 balls, flatten each ball with palm of hand**
3. **Heat a cast iron skillet with ghee over medium heat**
4. **Cook for 2-3 minutes remove and serve**

Chapter 30. Smoothie Recipes

PEANUT BUTTER COOKIES

Serves: *12*
Prep Time: *10*   Minutes
Cook Time: *30*   Minutes
Total Time: *40*   Minutes

INGREDIENTS

- 1 cup peanut butter (no sugar added)
- 1 tsp vanilla
- 1 tsp baking powder
- ½ tsp salt
- ½ cup keto sweetener such as Swerve, monk fruit sweetener or use stevia to taste
- 1 egg

DIRECTIONS

1. Preheat oven to 325 F
2. Cream together all ingredients
3. Refrigerate for 15-20 minutes
4. Roll dough into balls and place on a parchment paper lined baking sheet
5. Bake for 12-15 minutes

BUTTERY KETO CREPES

Serves: **2**

Prep Time:	**10**	Minutes
Cook Time:	**10**	Minutes
Total Time:	**20**	Minutes

INGREDIENTS

- 3 eggs
- ½ tsp vanilla extract
- ½ tsp cinnamon
- 3 oz cream cheese
- 2 tsp sweetener
- 2 tablespoons butter

DIRECTIONS

1. In a blender place all the ingredients and blend until smooth
2. In a buttered, hot skillet, pour batter and cook each crepe for 1-2 minutes per side or until ready
3. Remove and top with defrosted frozen berries and the defrosted juice.

Chapter 30. Smoothie Recipes

KETO LEMON FAT BOMBS

Serves: *4*
Prep Time: *10*   Minutes
Cook Time: *10*   Minutes
Total Time: *20*   Minutes

INGREDIENTS

- ½ cup coconut oil
- 3 tablespoons butter
- 3 oz cream cheese
- 2 tsp lemon juice
- 2 tsp sugar substitute such as monk fruit sweetener or Swerve

DIRECTIONS

1. **Place all ingredients in a mixing bowl and mix thoroughly**
2. **Spoon 1-2 tablespoons into two - four cupcake holders and freeze**
3. **Remove and serve**
4. **Recipe can be doubled for more servings**

PEANUT BUTTER BALLS

Serves: **4**
Prep Time: **10**   Minutes
Cook Time: **30**   Minutes
Total Time: **40**   Minutes

INGREDIENTS

- **1 cup peanuts finely chopped**
- **1 cup peanut butter (unsweetened)**
- **1 cup powdered sweetener such as Swerve confectioner's sugar**
- **6 oz sugar free (with stevia) chocolate chips or dark chocolate high% cacao chips**

DIRECTIONS

1. **In a bowl mix peanut butter, sweetener, chopped peanuts, divide dough into 12 pieces and shape into balls and place on a wax paper**
2. **Melt chocolate in a bowl over a pot of simmering water**
3. **Dip each peanut butter ball in the chocolate and place back on the wax paper**
4. **Refrigerate and serve**

Chapter 30. Smoothie Recipes

NUT-FREE KETO BROWNIE

Serves: *8*
Prep Time: *10*   Minutes
Cook Time: *20*   Minutes
Total Time: *30*   Minutes

INGREDIENTS

- 5 eggs
- ¼ lb butter
- 2 oz unsweetened cocoa powder
- ½ tsp baking powder
- 2 tsp vanilla
- ¼ lb cream cheese
- 3 tablespoons Swerve sweetener

DIRECTIONS

1. Place all the ingredients in a bowl and blend until smooth
2. Pour mixture into an oiled baking dish
3. Bake at 325 F for 20 minutes
4. Remove, slice into squares and serve

Chapter 30. Smoothie Recipes

COFFEE SMOOTHIE

Serves: *1*
Prep Time: *5*   Minutes
Cook Time: *5*   Minutes
Total Time: *10*   Minutes

INGREDIENTS

- 5 oz cold coffee
- 3 oz heavy cream
- 3 oz almond milk, unsweetened
- 1 oz chocolate syrup, unsweetened
- 1 oz caramel syrup, unsweetened
- 1 tablespoon cocoa, unsweetened
- 12 oz ice

DIRECTIONS

1. In a blender place all the ingredients and blend until smooth
2. Pour in a glass and serve

Chapter 30. Smoothie Recipes

CHAI PUMPKIN SMOOTHIE

Serves: *1*
Prep Time: **5**   Minutes
Cook Time: **5**   Minutes
Total Time: **10**   Minutes

INGREDIENTS

- ¾ cup coconut milk, unsweetened
- 2 tablespoon pumpkin puree
- 1 tablespoon MCT oil
- 1 tsp chai tea
- 1 tsp vanilla extract
- ½ tsp pumpkin pie spice
- ½ frozen avocado

DIRECTIONS

1. In a blender, place all the ingredients and blend until smooth
2. Pour in a glass and serve

CASHEW SMOOTHIE

Serves: *1*
Prep Time: **5**   Minutes
Cook Time: **5**   Minutes
Total Time: **10**   Minutes

INGREDIENTS

- **1 cup cashew milk, unsweetened**
- **1 tablespoon MCT oil**
- **1 tablespoon any nut butter**
- **1 tsp maca powder**
- **1 handful ice**

DIRECTIONS

1. **In a blender, place all the ingredients and blend until smooth**
2. **Pour in a glass and serve**

Chapter 30. Smoothie Recipes

BREAKFAST SMOOTHIE

Serves: *1*
Prep Time: **5** Minutes
Cook Time: **5** Minutes
Total Time: **10** Minutes

INGREDIENTS

- ½ cup almond milk, unsweetened
- ½ cup coconut milk, unsweetened
- ½ coconut yogurt, unsweetened
- ½ tsp powdered stevia
- 3 frozen strawberries

DIRECTIONS

1. In a blender, place all the ingredients and blend until smooth
2. Pour in a glass and serve

KETO MILKSHAKE SMOOTHIE

Serves: *1*
Prep Time: *5*   Minutes
Cook Time: *5*   Minutes
Total Time: *10*   Minutes

INGREDIENTS

- 6 oz plain almond milk, unsweetened
- 3 oz crushed ice
- 1 oz heavy whipping cream
- 1 oz frozen raspberries
- ¾ oz Swerve sweetener
- ½ oz cream cheese

DIRECTIONS

1. In a blender, place all the ingredients and blend until smooth
2. Pour in a glass and serve

Chapter 30. Smoothie Recipes

AVOCADO SMOOTHIE

Serves: *1*
Prep Time: *5*   Minutes
Cook Time: *5*   Minutes
Total Time: *10*   Minutes

INGREDIENTS

- ½ avocado
- 2 tablespoons cocoa powder, unsweetened
- 2/3 cup coconut milk, unsweetened
- ½ cup crushed ice
- ½ cup water
- Pinch of salt
- 1 tsp lime juice
- 4 stevia drops

DIRECTIONS

1. In a blender, place all the ingredients and blend until smooth
2. Pour in a glass and serve

COLLAGEN SMOOTHIE

Serves: *1*

Prep Time:	*5*	Minutes
Cook Time:	*5*	Minutes
Total Time:	*10*	Minutes

INGREDIENTS

- **4 ice cubes**
- **½ avocado**
- **1 scoop chocolate collagen powder**
- **1 tablespoon chia seeds, ground**
- **1 tablespoon almond butter, unsweetened**
- **¾ cup heavy whipping cream**
- **1 cup water**

DIRECTIONS

1. **In a blender place all the ingredients and blend until smooth**
2. **Pour in a glass and serve**

Chapter 30. Smoothie Recipes

FAT BOMB SMOOTHIE

Serves: *1*
Prep Time: *5*   Minutes
Cook Time: *5*   Minutes
Total Time: *10*   Minutes

INGREDIENTS

- 1/2 avocado
- 1 scoop collagen powder
- 1 tablespoon cacao powder
- 1 cup almond milk, unsweetened
- 4 drops stevia
- 1 cup ice

DIRECTIONS

1. In a blender place all the ingredients and blend until smooth
2. Pour in a glass and serve

CINNAMON SMOOTHIE

Serves: *1*
Prep Time: **5**   Minutes
Cook Time: **5**   Minutes
Total Time: **10**   Minutes

INGREDIENTS

- ½ cup coconut milk, full fat
- ½ cup water
- 2 ice cubes
- 1 tablespoon coconut oil
- ½ tsp ground cinnamon
- 1 tablespoon chia seeds, ground
- ½ cup vanilla protein powder (unsweetened)

DIRECTIONS

1. In a blender, place all the ingredients and blend until smooth
2. Pour in a glass and serve

Chapter 30. Smoothie Recipes

TROPICAL SMOOTHIE

Serves: *1*
Prep Time: *5*   Minutes
Cook Time: *5*   Minutes
Total Time: *10*   Minutes

INGREDIENTS

- ½ tsp banana extract
- ½ tsp blueberry extract
- ½ tsp mango extract
- 5 stevia drops
- 1 tablespoon coconut oil
- ½ cup sour cream
- Ice cubes
- ¾ cup coconut milk

DIRECTIONS

1. In a blender, place all the ingredients and blend until smooth
2. Pour in a glass and serve

Section VII: The Ketogenic Key – Concluding Thoughts

Wow! If you're at the end of this book and have read it all, well, congratulations to you – that was a lot of content! We hope you are now well versed on how the Ketogenic Key lifestyle can improve your physical, mental, and emotional health, as well as optimize your performance at pretty much everything in life!

Ketones and ketogenic therapies are here to stay, and we encourage you to try them and see how they make you feel and perform, and experience ketosis for yourself. Whether you choose to commit to the diet, or try boosting low-carb nutrition with ketone supplements, intermittent fasting, and exercise, is up to you. We would urge you to try it all, ideally in combination, because each method we describe has its own unique benefits and together they are incredibly powerful! Every person and their body is different, and will respond differently to the techniques we've described. So some experimentation is encouraged, coupled with testing your ketone levels, to see what works best for you.

The bottom line is that after this book is published, there will be more research, more clinical patient data, and more anecdotal data by people who took the step of believing and trying ketogenic therapies. Our goal with The Ketogenic Key was to discuss the importance and health benefits of ketogenic nutrition, as well go beyond that to show additional methods that may enhance and increase your ability to achieve and maintain a therapeutic level of ketosis, and allow you to experience the health benefits that ketones, especially beta-hydroxybutyrate, can have on your body and brain.

You have a choice right now. You're probably reading this book because you're curious about keto. So, choose health! Choose the Ketogenic Key lifestyle and see how much better you feel after

Section VII

experiencing the amazing state of ketosis by using any or all of methods we've laid out for you!

SECTION VIII: RESEARCH –
ANNOTATED SELECTED REFERENCES

Dear Readers:
We, the authors, are very scientifically minded in our approach to writing this book, and made extensive use of the medical and scientific literature around ketosis, ketone bodies, the ketogenic diet, fasting, exercise, nutrition, and exogenous ketone supplementation. We know, however, that research articles can sometimes be difficult to find, read, decipher, and understand – so we're doing the work for you!

This "Research" section contains selected references, which we've annotated with summaries and what we believe are the relevant key takeaways. We hope you will find this more useful than a long list of scientific citations whose titles do not always reflect or explain the conclusions of the study or literature review.

It's important to point out that as of this writing, there is a MASSIVE amount of research in process that has yet to be published, but will certainly come out in the next 1-2 years, and we expect even more conclusive, extensive and iron-clad scientific validation of the concepts and recommendations we are making in The Ketogenic Key.

We are starting with a group of papers that are some of what we consider to be of "Key" importance, as well as our favorites as science and research geeks, but have grouped most by topic area. We hope that you will find this to be an invaluable resource to study and share that reinforces and validates the underlying science and biology of ketones and ketosis!

Sincerely,
Dr. Lori and Steve

SECTION VIII

"KEY" STUDIES (And Some of Our Personal Favorites)

Veech RL. The therapeutic implications of ketone bodies: the effects of ketone bodies in pathological conditions: ketosis, ketogenic diet, redox states, insulin resistance and mitochondrial metabolism. *Prostaglandins Leukot Essent Fatty Acids.* 2004; 70:309-19.
https://www.sciencedirect.com/science/article/abs/pii/S0952327803002217
This early pivotal paper by keto pioneer Dr. Richard Veech (who passed away in early 2020) pointed out the potential therapeutic benefits of ketosis ketone bodies, especially beta-hydroxybutyrate, for three areas in particular: 1) diseases of substrate inefficiency (glucose hypometabolism) or insulin resistance; 2) diseases resulting from free radical damage; and 3) disease resulting from hypoxia (low oxygen). The article highlighted the direct metabolic effects of ketones as well as the higher energy derived from BHB compared to glucose. This article was part of a special issue that looked at the health implications of ketosis and ketone metabolism and set the groundwork for much of the research to come over the next 15+ years.

Myette-Cote E, Caldwell HG, Ainslie PN, et al. A ketone monoester drink reduces the glycemic response to an oral glucose challenge in individuals with obesity: a randomized trial. *Am J Clin Nutrition.* 2019; 110(6):1491-1501.
https://academic.oup.com/ajcn/article-abstract/110/6/1491/5585428
This well designed clinical trial showed that drinking a ketone monoester supplement before ingesting glucose resulted in better blood glucose stability in obese patients. This is important because it shows the potential for ketone supplements to aid in the control of blood sugar, especially in obese people who have diabetes, pre-diabetes, and insulin resistance.

Paoli A, Rubini A, Volek JS, Grimaldi KA. Beyond weight loss: a review of the therapeutic uses of very-low-carbohydrate (ketogenic) diets. *Eur J Clin Nutrition.* 2013; 67:789-96.
https://www.nature.com/articles/ejcn2013116
Hands down one of the most comprehensive and promising reviews in the literature. It assesses and comments on the weight of evidence for multiple therapeutic uses of low-carb ketogenic diets. It noted STRONG EVIDENCE for: (1) weight loss, (2) cardiovascular disease, (3) type 2 diabetes, and (4) Epilepsy. EMERGING EVIDENCE: (1) acne, (2) cancer, (3) polycystic ovary syndrome (PCOS), (4) neurologic diseases including Alzheimer's, Parkinson's, traumatic brain injury, ALS and more, and (5) respiratory function
It's important to note that this review is from 2013 – there has been significant numbers of new studies on ketosis, ketogenesis, the ketogenic diet, and ketone supplementation in the years since then, and we hope another equally comprehensive review of the literature will be done soon.

Youm YH, Nguyen KY, Grant RW, et al. The ketone metabolite β-hydroxybutyrate blocks NLRP3 inflammasome-mediated inflammatory disease. *Nature Medicine.* 2015; 21(3):263-269.
https://www.nature.com/articles/nm.3804
An excellent study published in *Nature Medicine,* one of the most prestigious scientific medical journals. A press release from Yale noted "the researchers described how beta-hydroxybutyrate (BHB) directly inhibits NLRP3, which is part of a complex set of proteins called the inflammasome. The inflammasome drives the inflammatory response in several disorders including autoimmune diseases, type 2 diabetes, Alzheimer's disease, atherosclerosis, and auto-inflammatory disorders. These findings are important because endogenous metabolites like BHB that block the NLRP3 inflammasome could be relevant against many inflammatory diseases…." The press release can be read in full here:
https://news.yale.edu/2015/02/16/anti-inflammatory-mechanism-dieting-and-fasting-revealed

Feinman RD, Pogozelski WK, Astrup A, et al. Dietary carbohydrate restriction as the first approach to diabetes management. *Nutrition.* 2015; 31(1):1-13.
https://www.sciencedirect.com/science/article/pii/S0899900714003323
This seminal study reviews evidence and makes clear-cut recommendations for carbohydrate restriction as the first approach in diabetes management. The authors note "such diets reliably reduce high blood glucose" and that "carbohydrate-restricted diets reduce or eliminate the need for medication." They also note "there are no side effects comparable with those seen in intensive pharmaceutical treatment."
We, the authors of this book, do not understand why this has not been widely adopted by healthcare systems, nutritionists and dieticians, and physicians, many of whom still cling to and communicate outdated dogma about low carb nutrition.

Goldberg EL, Molony RD, Kudo E, et al. Ketogenic diet activates protective γδ T cell responses against influenza virus infection. *Science Immunology.* 2019; 4 (41):eaav2026.
https://immunology.sciencemag.org/content/4/41/eaav2026
This study found that mice on a high-fat, low-carb ketogenic diet conferred immune response protection to influenza infection. They found that the ketogenic diet promoted the expansion of γδ T cells in the lungs and enhancing antiviral resistance. What was also interesting is that they also had study groups on a high-fat and high-carb diet, and they also provided a chemical ketone substrate supplement to some, and neither of those provided the specific protection, showing that this expansion of γδ T cells required metabolic adaptation to a ketogenic diet.

Volek J, Phinney SD. The art and science of low carbohydrate living: an expert guide to making the life-saving benefits of carbohydrate restriction sustainable and enjoyable. Lexington KY: Beyond Obesity. 2011; 1-302. https://www.amazon.com/Art-Science-Low-Carbohydrate-Living/dp/0983490708

This book is a phenomenal resource by two of the top minds in the low-carb and keto nutrition field. A must-read!

From Amazon: "Carbohydrate restricted diets are commonly practiced but seldom taught. As a result, doctors, dietitians, nutritionists, and nurses may have strong opinions about low carbohydrate dieting, but in many if not most cases, these views are not grounded in science. Now, whether you are a curious healthcare professional or just a connoisseur of diet information, two New York Times best selling authors provide you with the definitive resource for low carbohydrate living. Doctors Volek and Phinney share over 50 years of clinical experience using low carbohydrate diets, and together they have published more than 200 research papers and chapters on the topic. Particularly in the last decade, much has been learned about the risks associated with insulin resistance (including but not limited to metabolic syndrome, hypertension, and type-2 diabetes), and how this condition is far better controlled by carbohydrate restriction than with drugs."

Blaak EE, Antoine J-M, Benton D, et al. Impact of postprandial glycaemia on health and prevention of disease. *Obes Rev.* 2012; 13(10):923-984. https://www.ncbi.nlm.nih.gov/pmc/articles/PMC3494382/

This study looked at postprandial blood glucose spikes (blood sugar spikes after eating), because they are implicated in the development of metabolic diseases such as diabetes, obesity, and cardiovascular disease. They also increase oxidative stress and inflammation, and are linked to detriments in cognition and exercise capacity and performance. This review underscores the health implications of repeated blood sugar spikes – more reason to maintain a low-carb, low-sugar lifestyle!

Han Y-M, Ramprasath T, Zou M-H. -hydroxybutyrate and its metabolic effects of age-associated pathology. Exp Mol Med. 2020; April 8. DOI: https://doi.org/10.1038/s12276-020-0415-z
https://www.nature.com/articles/s12276-020-0415-z

This excellent review article was published under the prestigious Nature Publishing Group umbrella. It reviews a lot of animal and human studies as well as lab research to look at how ketones impact age-related disease and conditions. The abstract of this study really sums it up best:

> *"Aging is a universal process that renders individuals vulnerable to many diseases. Although this process is irreversible, dietary modulation and caloric restriction are often considered to have antiaging effects. Dietary modulation can increase and maintain circulating ketone bodies, especially β-hydroxybutyrate (β-HB), which is one of the most abundant ketone bodies in human circulation. Increased β-HB has been reported to prevent or improve the symptoms of various age-associated diseases.*

Indeed, numerous studies have reported that a ketogenic diet or ketone ester administration alleviates symptoms of neurodegenerative diseases, cardiovascular diseases, and cancers. Considering the potential of β-HB and the intriguing data emerging from in vivo and in vitro experiments as well as clinical trials, this therapeutic area is worthy of attention. In this review, we highlight studies that focus on the identified targets of β-HB and the cellular signals regulated by β-HB with respect to alleviation of age-associated ailments."

Puchalska P, Crawford P. Multi-dimensional roles of ketone bodies in fuel metabolism, signaling, and therapeutics. Cell Metab. 2017; 25(2):262-284. https://www.ncbi.nlm.nih.gov/pmc/articles/PMC5313038/
Another phenomenal review that points out the multi-faceted role that ketones play in the human body as a fuel source, metabolic influencer, signaling metabolite, and potential therapeutic agent. Much like the article cited previously, the abstract of this article really sums it up nicely:

"Ketone body metabolism is a central node in physiological homeostasis. In this review, we discuss how ketones serve discrete fine-tuning metabolic roles that optimize organ and organism performance in varying nutrient states, and protect from inflammation and injury in multiple organ systems. Traditionally viewed as metabolic substrates enlisted only in carbohydrate restriction, recent observations underscore the importance of ketone bodies as vital metabolic and signaling mediators when carbohydrates are abundant. Complementing a repertoire of known therapeutic options for diseases of the nervous system, prospective roles for ketone bodies in cancer have arisen, as have intriguing protective roles in heart and liver, opening therapeutic options in obesity-related and cardiovascular disease. Controversies in ketone metabolism and signaling are discussed to reconcile classical dogma with contemporary observations."

KETONES AND THE BRAIN: NEUROLOGIC BENEFITS

E. Deans, MD. "Your Brain On Ketones. How a high-fat diet can help the brain work better." *Psychology Today.* April 11, 2011. https://www.psychologytoday.com/us/blog/evolutionary-psychiatry/201104/your-brain-ketones
This article in *Psychology Today* discusses the benefits of a high-fat diet on cognition, neurologic diseases, and psychiatric disorders.

Safstrom CE, Rho JM. The ketogenic diet as a treatment paradigm for diverse neurological disorders. *Front Pharmacol.* 2012; 3:59.
https://www.ncbi.nlm.nih.gov/pmc/articles/PMC3321471/
This excellent review article summarizes the evidence and science and looks at how the ketogenic diet could be used to treat a number of neurologic conditions. Topics discussed include ketones for neuroprotection, epilepsy, aging, Alzheimer's disease, Parkinson's disease, ALS, cancer, stroke, mitochondrial disorders, brain trauma and TBI, psychiatric disorders such as depression, autism, migraines and more. A great look at the emerging data back in 2012, much of which is being implemented and researched further at the time of this book's writing.
You can read a great review of the study about the ketogenic diet for Alzheimer's disease here:
Ede G. Ketogenic diet promising for mild Alzheimer's disease. *Psychology Today.* March 31, 2018.
https://www.psychologytoday.com/us/blog/diagnosis-diet/201803/ketogenic-diet-promising-mild-alzheimers-disease

Gasior M, Rogawski MA, Hartman AL. Neuroprotective and disease modifying effects of the ketogenic diet. *Behav Pharmacol.* 2006; 17(5-6):431-439.
https://www.ncbi.nlm.nih.gov/pmc/articles/PMC2367001/
This outstanding review notes that a recent clinical study had raised the possibility that the ketogenic diet may confer long-lasting therapeutic benefits for patients with epilepsy. In addition, uncontrolled clinical trials and studies in animal models showed that the ketogenic diet can provide symptomatic and disease-modifying activity in a broad range of neurodegenerative disorders including Alzheimer's disease and Parkinson's disease, and may also be protective in traumatic brain injury and stroke. These observations are supported by studies in animal models and isolated cells that show that ketone bodies, especially β-hydroxybutyrate, confer neuroprotection against diverse types of cellular injury. This review summarizes the experimental, epidemiological and clinical evidence indicating that the ketogenic diet could have beneficial effects in a broad range of brain disorders characterized by the death of neurons. Although the mechanisms are not yet well defined, it is plausible that neuroprotection results from enhanced neuronal energy reserves, which improve the ability of

neurons to resist metabolic challenges, and possibly through other actions including antioxidant and anti-inflammatory effects.

Broom GM, Shaw IC, Rucklidge JJ. The ketogenic diet as a potential treatment and prevention strategy for Alzheimer's disease. *Nutrition.* 2019; 60:118-121. https://www.sciencedirect.com/science/article/pii/S0899900718302764 This study discusses the fact that impaired brain glucose metabolism and amyloid B plaques are associated with Alzheimer's disease, and looked at ketones due to their ability to provide an alternative fuel and metabolic precursor to glucose in the brain. They also hypothesize that ketogenic diets may reduce amyloid plaques and reverse their neurotoxicity.

Murphy P, Likhodii S, Nylen K, Burnham WM. Antidepressant properties of the ketogenic diet. *Biol Psych.* 2004; 56(12):981-983. https://www.biologicalpsychiatryjournal.com/article/S0006-3223(04)01006-6/fulltext This study on rats sought to shed light on a hypothesis about the ketogenic diet, which has been used to treat epilepsy and seizures. The hypothesis noted that individuals with epilepsy often have behavioral problems and deficits in attention and cognitive function, and the ketogenic diet has been found to help those issues and serve as a mood stabilizer. So they tested rats and found that the rats on the ketogenic diet spent less time being immobile and were less likely to exhibit "behavioral despair." Thus they concluded that the ketogenic diet might have anti-depressive qualities.

Palmer CM. Ketogenic diet in the treatment of schizoaffective disorder: two case studies. *Schizophrenia Research.* 2017; 189:208-209. https://www.sciencedirect.com/science/article/pii/S0920996417300634 An interesting case study of two patients who were treated with the ketogenic diet and were able to stop medications and were in remission. In fact the author wrote a piece in *Psychology Today* discussing the cases and the potential of the ketogenic diet in this disorder: https://www.psychologytoday.com/us/blog/advancing-psychiatry/201904/chronic-schizophrenia-put-remission-without-medication

Napoli E, Dueñas N, Giulivi C. Potential therapeutic use of the ketogenic diet in autism spectrum disorders. *Front Pediatr.* 2014; 2:69. https://www.ncbi.nlm.nih.gov/pmc/articles/PMC4074854/ This literature review discusses how the ketogenic diet has been used for epilepsy and other disorders, and has been advocated for use in a number of neurologic disorders, including autism spectrum disorders. They cite studies showing benefit, and discuss the potential mechanisms of how the ketogenic diet, and ketones, may help autism spectrum disorders, especially in terms of how better energy, mitochondrial function, and neurotransmitter management caused by ketones, may influence behavioral symptoms.

Lee RWY, Corley MJ, Pang A, et al. A modified ketogenic gluten-free diet with MCT improves behavior in children with autism spectrum disorder. *Physiol Behav.* 2018; 188:205-211.
https://www.ncbi.nlm.nih.gov/pmc/articles/PMC5863039/
A recent registered clinical trial (https://clinicaltrials.gov/ct2/show/NCT02477904) in 15 children in Honolulu that combined a ketogenic diet with MCT oil supplementation showed significant improvement in their core autism features, especially social affective components (fear, anxiety, and imitation).

Kashiwaya Y, Takeshima T, Mori N et al. D-B-Hydroxybutyrate protects neurons in models of Alzheimer's and Parkinson's disease. *PNAS.* 2000; 97(10):5440-5444.
https://www.pnas.org/content/97/10/5440.short
An interesting study that looked at brain energy metabolism as well as mitochondrial function. These authors had previously shown that ketone bodies could correct defects in heart muscle cell mitochondria energy generation. This study showed that ketone bodies protected neurons in the brain, and they hypothesize that ketones may play a therapeutic role in some of the most common forms of human neurodegeneration, including Alzheimer's disease and Parkinson's disease.

Vanitallie TB, Nonas C, Di Rocco A, et al. Treatment of Parkinson disease with diet-induced hyperketonemia: a feasibility study. *Neurology.* 2005; 64(4):728-730.
https://www.ncbi.nlm.nih.gov/pubmed/15728303
One published clinical study tested the effects of the ketogenic diet on symptoms of Parkinson's disease, and found that in a small cohort of 5 patients, the Unified Parkinson's Disease Rating Scale scores improved in all 5 during the time of elevated blood ketones.

Prins M, Matsumoto J. The collective therapeutic potential of cerebral ketone metabolism in traumatic brain injury. *J Lipid Res.* 2014; 55(12):2450-2457.
https://www.ncbi.nlm.nih.gov/pmc/articles/PMC4242438/
This study discusses how traumatic brain injury results in impaired and depressed glucose metabolism in the brain, from a number of factors including free radical production, ATP decreases, DNA damage and inhibition of key glycolytic enzymes. Because of this, glucose becomes an unfavorable energy substrate. The authors note that ketone bodies (especially beta-hydroxybutyrate) are the only known natural alternative fuel source to glucose for cerebral energy metabolism. They discuss how pre- and post-injury implementation of the ketogenic diet has demonstrated improved structural and functional outcome in traumatic brain injury models, concussion models, and spinal cord injury. They call for further clinical studies to identify the best method for infusing ketones in the postinjury

brain, as well as to validate the neuroprotective effects of ketogenic therapy in humans.

Fan, S. The fat-fueled brain: unnatural or advantageous? MIND Guest Blog. *Scientific American.* October 1, 2013. https://blogs.scientificamerican.com/mind-guest-blog/the-fat-fueled-brain-unnatural-or-advantageous/

Walker N. Can the ketogenic diet treat schizophrenia, anxiety, and depression? *Reports Healthcare.* April 23, 2018. https://reportshealthcare.com/12790/can-ketogenic-diet-treat-schizophrenia-anxiety-and-depression/

SECTION VIII

COGNITIVE FUNCTION
(Alzheimer's Disease, Dementia and Cognitive Impairment)

Mujica-Parodi LR, Amgalan A, Sultan SF, et al. Diet modulates brain network stability, a biomarker for brain aging, in young adults. *PNAS.* 2020; 3:201913042 DOI:10.1073/pnas.1913042117.
https://www.pnas.org/content/early/2020/03/02/1913042117/tab-article-info
This landmark study in humans was performed because epidemiologic studies have suggested that insulin-resistance accelerates progression of age-related cognitive impairment, which has been linked to glucose hypometabolism as well as an energy "gap" between what the brain needs, and what the body can supply (typically in glucose), a gap that is 7% in normal people and increases with age. The researchers looked at brain function and activity in patients before and after a ketogenic diet, as well as before and after consuming a ketone supplement vs a glucose supplement (and a ketone + glucose supplement). The results showed that the brain networks were destabilized by glucose, and stabilized by ketones, regardless of whether ketosis was achieved by diet or by supplementation. It also showed that the brain will take up ketones even when there is glucose consumed with it. Ketone utilization increases available energy and therefore may protect the aging brain. Because ketones are a high-yield fuel, they also help fill the brain energy gap.
Here is a great press release from the institution where the lead author works:
https://news.stonybrook.edu/newsroom/study-shows-low-carb-diet-may-prevent-reverse-age-related-effects-within-the-brain/

Crane PK, Walker R, Hubbard RA, et al. Glucose levels and risk of dementia. *N Engl J Med.* 2013; 369(6):540-48.
https://www.nejm.org/doi/full/10.1056/NEJMoa1215740
Important work establishing that higher glucose levels may be a risk factor for dementia, even among non-diabetics. The link between diabetes and higher incidence of dementia has been established, but this paper went beyond that to show it also is a potential risk in persons without diabetes. Higher levels of glucose may have damaging effects on the aging brain. This is significant because it emphasizes the importance of controlling blood glucose levels even when you are not diabetic – chronic elevated glucose may put you at risk for dementia and Alzheimer's disease.

De la Monte SM, Wands JR. Alzheimer's disease is type 3 diabetes – Evidence reviewed. *J Diabetes Sci and Tech.* 2008; 2(6): 1101-13.
https://journals.sagepub.com/doi/abs/10.1177/193229680800200619
An excellent literature and evidence review noting that 1) Type 2 diabetes causes brain insulin resistance, oxidative stress and cognitive impairment; 2)

the subsequent brain disturbances in brain insulin and insulin-like growth factor could account for the classic Alzheimer's brain lesions; 3) experimental models of brain diabetes share many characteristics with Alzheimer's disease including impaired brain energy (glucose) metabolism; and 4) that experimental brain diabetes was treatable with insulin sensitizer agents. This caused the authors to conclude that "Type 3 Diabetes" accurately reflects the fact that Alzheimer's disease represents a form of diabetes that selectively involves the brain.

Taylor MK, Sullivan DK, Mahnken JD, et al. Feasibility and efficacy data from a ketogenic diet intervention in Alzheimer's disease. *Alzheimer's Dementia Translational Res Clin Interventions*. 2018; 4:28-36. https://www.sciencedirect.com/science/article/pii/S2352873717300707 This study sought to assess the feasibility and cognitive effects of a ketogenic diet in patients with Alzheimer's disease with a pilot study. In this study, a group with mild impairment showed measurable improvement in cognitive function shown by results of the Alzheimer's Disease Assessment Scale scoring. Interestingly, these improved scores diminished after discontinuing the diet for 1 month.

Reger MA, Henderson ST, Hale C, et al. Effects of beta-hydroxybutyrate on cognition in memory-impaired adults. *Neurobiol Aging*. 2004; 25(3):311-14. https://www.ncbi.nlm.nih.gov/pubmed/15123336 A seminal randomized, controlled study on blood ketone levels and cognition. They studied 20 patients with Alzheimer's disease or mild cognitive impairment who consumed a drink containing MCTs (which convert easily to ketones) or a placebo. Significant increases in beta-hydroxybutyrate were observed 90 minutes after consumption of the MCT drink. Those who consumed the drink showed improvement in certain cognitive tests, prompting the authors to call for more research into the potential therapeutic benefits of increased ketone body blood concentrations.

Hoyer S. Abnormalities of glucose metabolism in Alzheimer's disease. *Ann NY Acad Sci.*1991; 640:53-8. https://www.ncbi.nlm.nih.gov/pubmed/1776759 This paper showed that the predominant disturbance in Alzheimer's is a significant reduction in cerebral glucose utilization, which caused a drastic loss of brain energy in all patients studied. This paper is significant for establishing that impaired glucose metabolism in the brain is a hallmark of Alzheimer's disease and dementia.

Cunnane SC, Courchesne-Loyer A, Vandenberghe C, et al. Can ketones help rescue brain fuel supply in later life? Implications for cognitive health during aging and the treatment of Alzheimer's disease. *Front Mol Neurosci.* 2016; 9(53).

SECTION VIII

https://www.ncbi.nlm.nih.gov/pmc/articles/PMC4937039/
An important study noting that because brain energy deficits are an important pre-symptomatic feature of Alzheimer's disease, and because brain uptake of ketones is not impacted in the brains of Alzheimer's patients, and that because interventions that raise ketone availability to the brain improve cognitive outcomes, the authors hypothesize that oral ketogenic supplements are a most promising means of achieving the goal of increasing brain energy metabolism.

Fortier M, Castellano CA, Croteau E, et al. A ketogenic drink improves brain energy and some measures of cognition in mild cognitive impairment. *Alzheimers Dement.* 2019; 15(5):625-634.
https://www.ncbi.nlm.nih.gov/pubmed/31027873
This is a blinded, randomized, placebo-controlled study of 52 subjects who were given a ketone drink or a placebo drink (no ketones) and researchers tested their cognitive performance at baseline vs 6 months later. Results showed that brain ketone metabolism increased by 230% in the group receiving the ketone drink. Measures of episodic memory, language, executive function, and processing speed improved in the ketone drink group vs baseline. This is significant because it showed that keeping ketones elevated into a therapeutic range helped brain function, even in people with cognitive impairment.

BETA-HYDROXYBUTYRATE AS A SIGNALING MOLECULE AND FIGHTER OF OXIDATIVE STRESS

Newman JC, Verdin E. Ketone bodies as signaling molecules. *Trends Endocrinol Metab.* 2014; 25(1): 42-52.
https://www.cell.com/trends/endocrinology-metabolism/fulltext/S1043-2760(13)00156-2
This report showed that ketone bodies have signaling functions as well as being a mobile source of energy. Ketone bodies inhibit histone deacetylases (which are implicated in aging) and control gene transcription. An important paper showing the anti-aging, metabolic modulation, and gene expression roles of ketones – which had mostly been considered as an alternative cellular fuel up until this time.

Newman JC, Verdin E. Beta-Hydroxybutyrate: Much more than a metabolite. *Diabetes Research Clin Practice.* 2014; 106(2):173-181.
https://www.diabetesresearchclinicalpractice.com/article/S0168-8227(14)00334-9/fulltext
Another study by Newman and Verdin in the journal *Diabetes Research and Clinical Practice* emphasizing the role of the ketone body BHB as having important cellular signaling roles both as an inhibitor of histone deacetylases (which regulate aging) as well as a ligand for cell receptors. BHB also produces downstream metabolic products that have signaling properties. They cite these aspects of cellular function and gene expression as having important implications for the pathogenesis and treatment of metabolic diseases, including type 2 diabetes.

Ruan HB, Crawford PA. Ketone bodies as epigenetic modifiers. *Curr Opn Clin Nutr Metab Care.* 2018; 21(4):260-266.
https://www.ncbi.nlm.nih.gov/pubmed/29697540
An excellent literature review that notes that direct regulation of gene expression in ketogenic states can be seen regardless of whether the ketogenic states are via diet, fasting, or exogenous ketone supplementation.

Koppel SJ, Swerdlow RH. Neuroketotherapeutics: A modern review of a century-old therapy. *Neurochem Int.* 2018; 117:113-125.
https://www.sciencedirect.com/science/article/abs/pii/S0197018617302279?via%3Dihub
This phenomenal review discusses neuroketotherapeutics, a class of bioenergetic medicine therapies that induce ketosis, which include MCT supplements, exogenous ketone supplements, fasting, strenuous exercise, the ketogenic diet and others. Per the abstract, "Extended experience reveals persons with epilepsy, especially pediatric epilepsy, benefit from ketogenic

diets".... "Data indicate neuroketotherapeutics enhance mitochondrial respiration, promoted neuronal long-term potentiation" and "attenuate oxidative stress, reduce inflammation, and alter protein post-translational modifications".... "Further studies of neuroketotherapeutics will enhance our understanding of ketone body molecular biology and reveal novel central nervous system therapeutic applications."

Youm YH, Nguyen KY, Grant RW, et al. The ketone metabolite β-hydroxybutyrate blocks NLRP3 inflammasome-mediate inflammatory disease. *Nature Medicine.* 2015; 21(3):263-9.
https://www.nature.com/articles/nm.3804
An excellent study published in *Nature Medicine*, one of the most prestigious medical scientific journals. A press release from Yale noted that "the researchers described how beta-hydroxybutyrate (BHB) directly inhibits NLRP3, which is part of a complex set of proteins called the inflammasome. The inflammasome drives the inflammatory response in several disorders including autoimmune diseases, type 2 diabetes, Alzheimer's disease, atherosclerosis, and auto-inflammatory disorders. These findings are important because endogenous metabolites like BHB that block the NLRP3 inflammasome could be relevant against many inflammatory diseases...." The press release can be read in full here:
https://news.yale.edu/2015/02/16/anti-inflammatory-mechanism-dieting-and-fasting-revealed

Shimazu T, Hirschey MD, Newman J, et al. Suppression of oxidative stress by β-hydroxybutyrate, an endogenous histone deacetylase inhibitor. *Science.* 2013; 339(6116):211-214.
https://science.sciencemag.org/content/339/6116/211.long
This study in the prestigious journal *Science* showed the administration of the ketone metabolite beta-hydroxybutyrate (BHB) by consuming an exogenous ketone supplement, or increasing levels in the body from fasting, were both effective at conferring substantial protection against oxidative stress in mice. In fact, it protected them from the toxic effects of oxidative stress-causing poison paraquat.

Settergren G, Lindblad BS, Persson B. Cerebral blood flow and exchange of oxygen, glucose, ketone bodies, lactate, pyruvate and amino acids in infants. *Acta Paediatr. Scand.* 1976; 65:343–353.
https://onlinelibrary.wiley.com/doi/abs/10.1111/j.1651-2227.1976.tb04896.x
This study from the 1970s showed that infants have a higher mean cerebral blood flow and greater uptake of ketone bodies than had been reported in adults, showing a possible mechanism for why the ketogenic diet is more effective in pediatric epilepsy patients than in adults. Another important concept supporting that ketones are not only an excellent fuel for the brain,

they may actually be the preferred fuel. It also showed how ketones easily cross the blood/brain barrier.

Adam PA, Raiha N, Rahiala EL, Kekomaki M. Oxidation of glucose and D-B-OH-butyrate by the early human fetal brain. *Acta Paediatr. Scand.* 1975; 64:17–24.
https://onlinelibrary.wiley.com/doi/10.1111/j.1651-2227.1975.tb04375.x
Another seminal study from the 1970s showing that both glucose and ketones support oxidative metabolism in the brain, and that beta-hydroxybutyrate is identified as a major potential alternate fuel that can replace glucose early in human development. This is a very important concept to understand, especially when combating the uninformed pseudo-nutritionists and dieticians who claim that carbohydrates are required by the body and brain and therefore must be consumed in quantities that would be detrimental to ketosis. The fact is, the body and brain do not need carbs because they can run just fine on ketones. For those bodily functions that do require glucose or glycogen, your body can produce glucose from protein and other substrates by the action of gluconeogenesis, so consuming carbohydrates in the diet is not necessary or required.

FAT LOSS, WEIGHT LOSS AND ANTI-OBESITY

World Health Organization. Health Topics: Obesity and Overweight. 2016.
http://www.who.int/en/news-room/fact-sheets/detail/obesity-and-overweight
A WHO statement noting that worldwide obesity has tripled since 1975, and citing statistics on global obesity.

Volek JS, Phinney SD, Forsythe CE, et al. Carbohydrate restriction has more favorable impact on the metabolic syndrome than a low fat diet. *Lipids.* 2009; 44(4):297-309.
https://aocs.onlinelibrary.wiley.com/doi/abs/10.1007/s11745-008-3274-2
This key study by Volek and Phinney, pioneers in studying low carb and ketogenic dieting, showed that carb restriction improved nearly every marker of cardiovascular disease as well as metabolic syndrome, with the authors noting that the results support the use of dietary carb restriction as an effective approach to improve metabolic syndrome and cardiovascular risk.

Malik VS, Hu FB. Popular weight-loss diets: from evidence to practice. *Nature Clin Pract Cardiovasc Med.* 2007; 4(1):34-41.
https://www.nature.com/articles/ncpcardio0726
An outstanding article from the Nature publishing group showing the superiority of low-carb diets over low-fat diets. The authors discuss the fact that obesity has become one of the leading public health concerns in many countries, and as a result there has been a rise in the popularity and use of various weight-loss diets. The authors note that low-carbohydrate diets are attractive because they promise rapid weight loss without having to count calories. Evidence indicates that low-carb diets could be better for weight loss than low-fat diets. They discuss the Mediterranean diet in depth including how it has been shown to improve cardiovascular risk factors and reduce risk of chronic diseases, although long-term studies have yet to be convincingly demonstrated.

Gomez-Arbelaez D, Bellido D, Castro AI, et al. Body composition changes after very-low-calorie ketogenic diet in obesity evaluated by 3 standardized methods. *J Clin Endocrinol Metab.* 2017; 102(2):488-498.
https://academic.oup.com/jcem/article/102/2/488/2972058
A comprehensive study published by The Endocrine Society in the *Journal of Clinical Endocrinology and Metabolism.* The authors looked at very low calorie ketogenic diets to assess the theory that much of the reported weight loss is due to muscle cannibalism. However, their conclusions showed that most of the weight loss was fat mass and visceral fat mass, whereas muscle mass and strength were preserved. This is an important study because it shows the effectiveness of the ketogenic diet at reducing overall fat mass, but especially

visceral fat (fat surrounding the organs) which is highly correlated with hypertension, high triglycerides, diabetes and even cancer. This study also cited 2 studies that showed benefit if the ketogenic diet after 1 and 2 years, showing its long-term effectiveness (that's important because critics often say the keto diet is not safe long-term nor sustainable long-term, which these studies prove to be not true – it is both safe and effective over long term studies).

NOTE: One thing that we, the authors of this book, want to point out is that many of the older studies discussed in this article used a very low calorie "starvation" diet to achieve ketosis – of course, we now know that you do not have to reduce calories to that level to achieve ketosis if you follow a well-formulated keto diet.

Moreno B, Bellido D, Sajoux I, et al. Comparison of a very low calorie ketogenic diet with a standard low-calorie diet in the treatment of obesity. *Endocrine.* 2014; 47(3):793-805.
https://www.ncbi.nlm.nih.gov/pubmed/24584583
This study showed that a ketogenic diet was both safe and effective after 1 year, again, showing that critics are mistaken when they claim the diet is neither safe nor sustainable long term. It is, and studies like this are proof.

Hallberg SJ, McKenzie AL, Williams PT, et al. Effectiveness and safety of a novel care model for the management of type 2 diabetes at 1 year: an open-label, non-randomized, controlled study. *Diabetes Ther.* 2018; 9:583–612.
https://link.springer.com/article/10.1007%2Fs13300-018-0373-9
This registered clinical trial (NCT02519309) of 349 adults with type 2 diabetes showed that a ketogenic diet that achieved nutritional ketosis with remote counseling and coaching resulted in 94% of users reducing or eliminating their need for insulin and metformin type drugs. They also lost weight and showed improvement in cardiovascular and other health markers.

Gibson AA, Seimon RV, Lee CMY, et al. Do ketogenic diets really suppress appetite? A systematic review and meta-analysis. *Obesity Reviews.* 2015; 6: 64–76.
https://www.ncbi.nlm.nih.gov/pubmed/25402637
This study showed that the ketogenic diet did, in fact, really suppress appetite in patients. This is significant because we know that many diets fail to work because people get hungrier during diets that require calorie and food restrictions. One of the very positive aspects of eating a high-fat diet like the ketogenic diet is that the fats satiate the dieter and help them feel full and less hungry, or hungry less often. In addition, these authors attribute some of the appetite suppressive effects to be a result of being in the state of ketosis – not just because they ate a lot of fat.

SECTION VIII

Hribal ML, Fiorentino TV, Sesti G. Role of C reactive protein (CRP) in leptin resistance. *Curr Pharm Des.* 2014; 20(4):609-615.
https://www.ncbi.nlm.nih.gov/pubmed/23688010
A study on inflammation and hunger hormones that showed that chronic elevation of C reactive protein (a marker of inflammation) in obese subjects worsens leptin resistance and endothelial dysfunction. This supports the theory of a negative cycle loop where inflammation present in obesity suppresses the hormone leptin, which signals your body to stop eating, and the resistance leads to continued overeating and inflammation, which further increases leptin resistance.

Sumithran P, Prendergast LA, Delbridge E, et al. Ketosis and appetite-mediating nutrients and hormones after weight loss. *Eur J Clin Nutr.* 2013; 67(7):759-764.
https://www.ncbi.nlm.nih.gov/pubmed/23632752
This study looked at how the ketogenic diet affected appetite. It's well documented that diet-induced weight loss of cutting back calories can lead to changes in appetite and satiety hormones that result in weight regain. These researchers put people on a ketogenic diet and then reintroduced foods, while testing levels of glucose, insulin, BHB, leptin, ghrelin and other GI hormones, and appetite. The results showed that the keto group lost weight (no surprise there) and that while in ketosis, their ghrelin (the "hunger hormone" that causes increases in appetite) was suppressed. So this study confirmed that keto helps reduce food cravings and suppresses appetite-stimulating hormones!

Nazish, N. How to eat keto the right way, according to a nutritionist. *Forbes.* August 31, 2018.
https://www.forbes.com/sites/nomanazish/2018/08/31/how-to-eat-keto-the-right-way-according-to-a-nutritionist/#2e843f892c5e

TYPE 2 DIABETES

Feinman RD, Pogozelski WK, Astrup A, et al. Dietary carbohydrate restriction as the first approach to diabetes management. *Nutrition.* 2015; 31(1):1-13. https://www.sciencedirect.com/science/article/pii/S0899900714003323
This seminal, multi-country study reviews evidence and makes clear-cut recommendations for carbohydrate restriction as the first approach in diabetes management. The authors state that "such diets reliably reduce high blood glucose" and that "carbohydrate-restricted diets reduce or eliminate the need for medication." They also state that "there are no side effects comparable with those seen in intensive pharmaceutical treatment."
We, the authors of this book, do not understand why this has not been widely adopted by healthcare systems, nutritionists and dieticians, and physicians, many of whom still cling to and communicate outdated dogma about low carb nutrition.
[Note: we repeated this from our favorites list in the beginning of this section because it's THAT important of a study.]

Centers for Disease Control and Prevention. Diabetes Statistics: National Diabetes Statistics Reports
https://www.cdc.gov/diabetes/data/statistics/statistics-report.html
National statistics on diabetes. Worth a look – it's shocking to see how much of our US population has diabetes!

Hammami MM. Book Review: Diabetes mellitus: A fundamental and clinical text. *Ann Saudi Med.* 1997;17:264.

van Zuuren EJ, Fedorowicz Z, Kuijpers T, Pijl H. Effects of low-carbohydrate- compared to low-fat-diet interventions on metabolic control in people with type 2 diabetes: a systematic review including GRADE assessments. *Am J Clin Nutrition.* 2018; 108(2):300-331.
https://academic.oup.com/ajcn/article/108/2/300/5051863
This large systematic review of multiple randomized controlled trials, which have the most desirable levels of evidence, compared the effects of dietary carb restriction vs fat restriction on markers of metabolic syndrome and quality of life in people with type 2 diabetes. The study showed that dietary carbohydrate restriction yielded slightly better metabolic control than reduction in fat.

Saltiel AR, Olevsky JM. Inflammatory mechanisms linking obesity and metabolic disease. *J Clin Invest.* 2017; 127:1-4.
https://www.jci.org/articles/view/92035

SECTION VIII

This article discusses the worldwide obesity epidemic, and what we currently know about obesity and inflammation, including: activation of the immune system in obesity; inflammation in diabetic islets, brain, liver, gut, and muscles; the role of inflammation in fibrosis and angiogenesis; the factors that contribute to the initiation of inflammation in obesity; and therapeutic approaches to modulate inflammation in obesity and metabolic syndrome.

Saslow LR, Daubenmier JJ, Moskowitz JT, et al. Twelve month outcomes of a randomized trial of moderate-carbohydrate vs very low carbohydrate diet in overweight adults with type 2 diabetes mellitus or prediabetes. *Nutrition Diabetes*. 2017; 7(12):304.
https://www.nature.com/articles/s41387-017-0006-9
This study published in the Nature group's journal *Nutrition & Diabetes,* showed that participants of the low-carb-ketogenic diet group reduce the use of their medication more than the group in a moderate carb diet, and showed greater reductions in A1c and weight.
More about this study can be found here:
https://blog.virtahealth.com/one-year-clinical-trial-outcomes-type-2-diabetes/

HEART DISEASE

Dehghan M, Mente A, Zhang X, et al. Associations of fats and carbohydrate intake with cardiovascular disease and mortality in 18 countries from five continents (PURE): a prospective cohort study. *Lancet.* 2017: 360(10107):2050-2062.
https://www.thelancet.com/journals/lancet/article/PIIS0140-6736(17)32252-3/fulltext
This prospective study looked at an epidemiologic cohort of 135,335 individuals using food frequency questionnaires. The study noted that higher carbohydrate intake was associated with an increased risk of total mortality. Higher total fat intake was associated with lower risk of total mortality. Higher saturated fat intake was associated with lower risk of stroke. Total fat and saturated and unsaturated fats were not significantly associated with risk of heart attack or cardiovascular disease mortality.
This study is significant because it refuted the conventional wisdom that fat causes higher incidence of heart disease and stroke mortality. Although it called for global dietary guidelines to be reconsidered in light of the findings, very little has changed in dietary recommendations, which still push a high-carb, low-fat dogma that has been disproven.

Nielsen R, Moller N, Gormsen LC, et al. Cardiovascular effects of treatment with the ketone body β-hydroxybutyrate in chronic heart failure patients. *Circulation.* 2019; 139:2129-2141.
https://www.ahajournals.org/doi/10.1161/CIRCULATIONAHA.118.036459
In patients with heart failure and reduced ejection fraction, infusion of the ketone body BHB increased cardiac output by 2L/min (40%) with an absolute improvement in left ventricular ejection fraction (8%). These effects were accompanied by vasodilation and stable systemic and pulmonary blood pressure. The authors concluded that this might represent a new treatment principle in patients with heart failure.

Bhanpuri NH, Hallberg SJ, Willliams PT, et al. Cardiovascular disease risk factor responses to a type 2 diabetes care model including nutritional ketosis induced by sustained carbohydrate restriction at 1 year: an open-label, non-randomized, controlled study. *Cardiovasc Diabetology.* 2018; 17(56).
https://cardiab.biomedcentral.com/articles/10.1186/s12933-018-0698-8
This article which included authors Phinney and Volek noted that a continuous care treatment including nutritional ketosis in patients with type 2 diabetes improve most biomarkers of cardiovascular disease risk after 1 year, including lipids, inflammation, and blood pressure.

Kolwicz Jr. SC, Airhart S, Tian R. Ketones step to the plate: A game changer for metabolic remodeling in heart failure? *Circulation.* 2016; 133:689-691.

https://www.ahajournals.org/doi/10.1161/CIRCULATIONAHA.116.021230
This editorial sheds light on the following two studies by Aubert and Bedi and colleagues.

Aubert G, Martin OJ, Horton JL et al. The failing heart relies on ketone bodies as a fuel. *Circulation.* 2016; 133:698-705.
https://www.ahajournals.org/doi/10.1161/CIRCULATIONAHA.115.017355
This study was prompted by evidence that shows that the failing heart is energy starved. During the development of heart failure, the heart's ability to use fatty acids (its chief fuel) is diminished. These researchers note that the failing heart resorts to using ketone bodies as a fuel source. Although the researchers are not sure if this is an adaptive response, they call for the need for further study, as this may delineate future therapeutic options.

Bedi Jr. KC, Snyder NW, Brandimarto J, et al. Evidence for intramyocardial disruption of lipid metabolism and increased myocardial ketone utilization in advanced human heart failure. *Circulation.* 2016; 133:706-716.
https://www.ahajournals.org/doi/10.1161/CIRCULATIONAHA.115.017545
Like the previous study, these researchers showed that in human heart failure patients, the body switches fuel sources from fatty acids or glucose to ketone bodies as an adaptive metabolic strategy.

Kearns CE, Schmidt LA, Glantz SA. Sugar industry and coronary heart disease research: a historical analysis of internal industry documents. *JAMA Intern Med.* 2016; 176(11):1680-1685.
https://jamanetwork.com/journals/jamainternalmedicine/article-abstract/2548255
This analysis of internal sugar industry documents showed that the sugar industry sponsored a research program in the 1960s and 70s that successfully cast doubt on the dangers of sugar (sucrose) and promoted fat as the dietary culprit in coronary heart disease. The authors called for policymaking committees to consider giving less weight to food industry-sponsored studies.

Malholtra A, Redberg RF, Meier P. Saturated fat does not clog the arteries: coronary heart disease is a chronic inflammatory condition, the risk of which can be effectively reduced from healthy lifestyle interventions. *Brit J Sports Med.* 2017; 51:1111-1112.
https://bjsm.bmj.com/content/51/15/1111.full
This editorial by renowned cardiologist Aseem Malholtra and colleagues discusses the inflammatory nature of coronary heart disease, pointing out that sugar and refined carbohydrates, not fats, are the key causes of multiple factors that lead to heart disease. They recommend a Mediterranean style diet high in vegetables, healthy fats and low in sugar and refined carbohydrates.

Gibas MK, Gibas KJ. Induced and controlled dietary ketosis as a regulator of obesity and metabolic syndrome pathologies. *Diabetes Metabolic Syndrome Clin Research Rev.* 2017; 11 (supplement 1):S385-S390.
https://www.sciencedirect.com/science/article/abs/pii/S1871402116303137
This study followed 30 patients randomized to 3 groups including one following a ketogenic diet with no exercise (vs a standard American diet with exercise and a standard American diet without exercise). The ketogenic diet group outperformed the other two groups for weight loss, body fat reduction, BMI, and A1c.
This study is significant because it showed that even without exercise, a ketogenic diet helps with multiple health markers compared to a standard American diet, even with exercise.

Strohle A, Hahn A. Diets of modern hunter-gathers vary substantially in their carbohydrate content depending on ecoenvironments: results from an ethnographic analysis. *Nutrition Research.* 2011; 31(6):429-435.
https://www.sciencedirect.com/science/article/pii/S0271531711000911?via%3Dihub
This study analyzed the diets of hunter-gatherers in different environments and found that regardless of where they lived, their intake of carbs was significantly lower than the amounts currently recommended for healthy humans.
This study is significant because we know that hunter-gatherers have low incidence of heart disease and most modern non-communicable diseases such as obesity, diabetes, and metabolic syndrome.

Kosinski C, Jornayvaz FR. Effects of ketogenic diets on cardiovascular risk factors: evidence from animal and human studies. *Nutrients.* 2017; 9(5):517.
https://www.ncbi.nlm.nih.gov/pmc/articles/PMC5452247/
This paper looked at human and animal studies to determine the long term efficacy and safety of ketogenic diets. Although somewhat controversial, the authors did conclude that the ketogenic diet might be associated with improvements in some cardiovascular risk factors. They authors claimed the effects are limited in time and there are some potential risks (we the authors of this book would argue more evidence has shown them to be sustainable long term as well as safe). However, some of the reviews cited show strong evidence for the benefits of the ketogenic diet.

Grynberg A, Demaison L. Fatty acid oxidation and the heart. *J Cardiovasc Pharmacol.* 2996; 28(suppl 1):S11-17.
https://www.ncbi.nlm.nih.gov/pubmed/8891866
An excellent review of how the heart uses fatty acids for energy and metabolism, and how it can switch from one fuel source to another in times of need or injury.

DIETARY INTERVENTIONS FOR HIGH BLOOD PRESSURE

Yancy WS, Westman EC, McDuffie JR, et al. A randomized trial of a low-carbohydrate diet vs Orlistat plus a low-fat diet for weight loss. *Arch Intern Med. 2010; 170(2):136-145.*
https://jamanetwork.com/journals/jamainternalmedicine/fullarticle/415539
This study in 146 patients compared a low-carb keto diet vs a low-fat diet combined with the weight-loss drug Orlistat (a lipase inhibitor that prevents the absorption of fats). In this particular study, not only was the keto diet alone as good as a low-fat diet combined with a weight loss drug, the patients on the keto diet also saw better results in reducing their blood pressure, which we believe is very significant for keto-curious people to know.

Pérez-Guisado J, Muñoz-Serrano A, Alonso-Moraga A. Spanish ketogenic Mediterranean diet: a healthy cardiovascular diet for weight loss. *Nutrition J.* 2008; 7:30.
https://doi.org/10.1186/1475-2891-7-30
This prospective study on 31 obese patients utilized a modified ketogenic diet with Spanish and Mediterranean characteristics that was particularly rich in olive oil, salad, fish, and red wine. Participants showed significant reductions in weight, BMI, blood pressure, and triglycerides, and showed greatly improved lipid profiles.

Park S, An J, Lee BK. Very-low-fat diets may be associated with increased risk of metabolic syndrome in the adult population. *Clinical Nutrition* 2016; 35(5): 1159-1167.
https://www.clinicalnutritionjournal.com/article/S0261-5614(15)00244-7/abstract
This cross-sectional study looked at more than 34,000 Korean patients who were tracked to see how fat intake correlated with prevalence of metabolic syndrome. The authors were surprised (but we are not!) to find that the prevalence of metabolic syndrome was significantly higher in the low fat diet group, even when fewer calories were consumed.

Appel LJ, Brands MW, Daniels SR, et al. Dietary approaches to prevent and treat hypertension a scientific statement from the American Heart Association. *Hypertension.* 2006; 47(2):296-308. https://www.ahajournals.org/doi/full/10.1161/01.HYP.0000202568.01167.B6
This statement on high blood pressure from the American Heart Association discusses weight loss as an effective way to lower blood pressure. They also discuss the DASH recommendations at length – (Dietary Approaches to Stop Hypertension). Some interesting things they note is that >75% of consumed salt comes from processed foods! They also note the blood pressure lowering affect of high potassium intake.

Most significant, however, was the comparison of the OmniHeart diet to the DASH diet, where they looked at different versions with various carb, protein, and fat consumption levels. What they found was that reducing carbs and replacing those calories with increased protein or fats showed greater reductions in blood pressure. We feel this is significant because it shows that lowering your carbs can lead to better blood pressure levels.

They also discussed studies that showed that high sugar consumption raises blood pressure.

Yoon SS, Burt V, Louis T, Carroll MD. Hypertension among adults in the United States, 2009-2010. *NCHS Data Brief.* 2012; 107:1-8. https://books.google.com/books?id=1551f1Ovxx8C
This data brief from the US Department of Health and Human Services at the CDC discusses key findings from the National Health and Nutrition Examination Survey of 2009-2010, including the prevalence (28.6%) and that 76% of those with hypertension were taking medication for it.

James PA, Oparil S, Carter BL, et al. 2014 evidence-based guideline for the management of high blood pressure in adults: report from the panel members appointed to the Eighth Joint National Committee (JNC 8). *JAMA.* 2014; 311(5):507-520. https://www.ncbi.nlm.nih.gov/pubmed/24352797
This guideline for treating hypertension sets the definition of "high blood pressure" at 140/90 and cites various pharmaceutical interventions to be used in different patient groups with various characteristics. This is important because recently the definition of high blood press was LOWERED – which of course means that millions more people can now be considered to have high blood pressure, and treated with medications. Interesting to note that this guideline is all about pharmacologic treatments. It contains no discussions of using diet or nutritional interventions to lower blood pressure. It does mention in almost in passing in its Conclusion section, noting that "the potential benefits of a healthy diet, weight control, and regular exercise cannot be overemphasized. These lifestyle treatments have the potential to improve BP control and even reduce medication needs. Although the authors of this hypertension guideline did not conduct and evidence review of lifestyle treatments in patients taking and not taking antihypertensive

medication, we support the recommendations of the 2013 Lifestyle Work Group."

Wright JT and the SPRINT Research Group. A randomized trial of intensive versus standard blood-pressure control. *N Engl J Med.* 2015; 373(22):2103-2116.
https://www.nejm.org/doi/full/10.1056/NEJMoa1511939
This study found that targeting a systolic blood pressure less than 120 mm Hg resulted in lower rates of fatal and nonfatal cardiovascular events and death. The authors also pointed out that trying to achieve a BP lower than 120 would likely require at least one additional medication in most patients, which would necessitate increased medication costs and clinic visits. The NIH eventually adopted this definition for national health standards.
It is significant because by lowering the baseline target for blood pressure, millions more people care considered to have high blood pressure, and therefore should be treated for it with medications. One estimate noted that it could mean an additional 8.6 million people who would "need" hypertension therapy.

CANCER

Cohen CW, Fontaine KR, Arend RC, et al. A ketogenic diet reduces central obesity and serum insulin in women with ovarian or endometrial cancer. *J Nutrition.* 2018;148(8):1253–1260.
https://academic.oup.com/jn/article/148/8/1253/5064353
This landmark article looks at cancer as a metabolic disease, hallmarked by cancer cells having a high metabolic preference (or requirement) for glucose, and that they may be vulnerable to conditions of glucose deprivation. Therefore, they studied the ketogenic diet vs the American Cancer Society diet on glucose and insulin levels in 73 female patients with either ovarian or endometrial cancer because both are strongly associated with obesity. Results showed that the ketogenic diet resulted in lower body fat, android fat, and visceral fat, as well as lower insulin and c-Peptide.
The authors concluded that "In aggregate, these finding suggest that the ketogenic diet creates a metabolic environment that is not supportive of cancer proliferation."

Hou Y, Zhou, M, Xie J, et al. High glucose levels promote the proliferation of breast cancer cells through GTPases. *Breast Cancer: Targets and Therapy.* 2017; 9:429-436.
https://www.ncbi.nlm.nih.gov/pubmed/28670141
High levels of glucose in the body, as well as diabetes, have been linked to an increase in cancer for years. But this study looked at how that link may take place. The authors demonstrated that high glucose levels in the body actually promoted the proliferation of breast cancer cells by stimulating various cellular growth factor receptors, as well as impacting cell signaling.

Poff AM, Ari C, Arnold P, Seyfried TN, D'Agostino DP. Ketone supplementation decreases tumor cell viability and prolongs survival of mice with metastatic cancer. *Int J Cancer.* 2014; 135(7):1711-1720.
https://onlinelibrary.wiley.com/doi/full/10.1002/ijc.28809
This eye-opening study on ketone supplementation in mice with metastatic cancer randomized mice to one of 4 treatments: (1) a standard diet, (2) a standard diet + 1,3-butanediol, (3) a standard diet + ketone supplement, or (4) a calorie restricted diet. Results showed that the group supplemented with ketones and the group supplemented with 1,3-butanediol both saw significant improvements in tumor growth (*i.e.,* less growth) as well as survival. In fact, the ketone group saw survival time increase by 69%. In addition, ketones were effective regardless of whether the group was consuming glucose or not (meaning it is the ketone bodies, not the diet, that is causing the effect).
This study is highly significant because it shows preliminary promise in animal studies that ketones may have as an adjuvant anti-cancer therapy.

Weber DD, Aminazdeh-Gohari S, Kofler B. Ketogenic diet in cancer therapy. *Aging.* 2018; 10(2):164-165.
https://www.ncbi.nlm.nih.gov/pmc/articles/PMC5842847/
This editorial in the journal *Aging* reviewed the literature and also the authors discussed their own research. They found that the growth of neuroblastoma (a type of brain cancer) was significantly reduced by a ketogenic diet. In addition, they reviewed studies on different types of cancer, and the results of those studies, pointing out that while in many types of cancer, the ketogenic diet has had an impact on slowing cancer cell growth, or has been to be effective when combined with adjuvant therapies like chemo and radiation, not all cancers have reacted that way. Therefore, it's important to note that some cancer types are impacted significantly by the ketogenic diet alone or in combination with other therapies, while other cancer types may not be as sensitive to it.

Tan-Shalaby JL, Carrick J, Edinger K, et al. Modified Atkins diet in advanced malignancies – final results of a safety and feasibility trial within the Veterans Affairs Pittsburgh Healthcare System. *Nutr Metab.* 2016; 13:52.
https://nutritionandmetabolism.biomedcentral.com/articles/10.1186/s12986-016-0113-y
These researchers studied 11 cancer patients to test the ketogenic diet's safety and feasibility in cancer patients across a variety of tumor types. Most notably, survival improved in some melanoma and lung cancer patients.

Caccialanza R, Cereda E, De Lorenzo F, et al on behalf of the AIOM-SINPE-FAVO Working Group. To fast, or not to fast before chemotherapy, that is the question. *BMC Cancer.* 2018; 18:337
https://bmccancer.biomedcentral.com/articles/10.1186/s12885-018-4245-5
This article from the "Debate" section of an open access cancer journal discusses some of the preliminary data on fasting and starvation-mimicking diets (which are also considered ketogenic) and chemotherapy. Although they point out some preliminary animal and human trials that show some benefits such as protecting healthy cells from chemotherapy, that it can activate other oncogenes in cancer cells and decrease cellular growth rates while increasing sensitivity to anti-mitotic drugs (drugs that keep cells from multiplying) and that some fasting-mimicking diets improved some health markers in patients. But the authors point out that fasting could increase the potential for malnutrition and muscle wasting in cancer patients who are already struggling to with their nutritional intake. Their conclusion is that the information has been too generalized and that it's too soon to make a definitive recommendation, and that there needs to be identification of a specific patient group and cancer type to do a meaningful study.

Caffa I, D'Agostino V, Damonte P, et al. Fasting potentiates the anticancer activity of tyrosine kinase inhibitors by strengthening MAPK signaling inhibition. *Oncotarget.* 2015; 6:11820-11832. https://doi.org/10.18632/oncotarget.3689
This laboratory cell study looked at the ability of starvation and calorie restriction to make chemotherapy drugs more effective. The authors noted that "here we report that starvation conditions increase the ability of commonly administered TKI's"…." to block cancer cell growth, to inhibit the mitogen-activated protein kinase (MAPK) signaling pathway, and to strengthen E2F-dependent transcription inhibition." They also noted several clinical trials currently studying fasting and fasting-mimicking diets in patients undergoing chemotherapy, and that preliminary data show that it can be safely introduced in patients, and they cited other studies showing a reduced risk of leukopenia (drop in white blood cells, which is a potential side effect of chemo in cancer patients). The lab studies on cells conducted by this group supported the potential positive effects of fasting and starvation-mimicking diets, and the authors called for additional clinical trials with patients.

Cheng CW, Adams GB, Perin L, et al. Prolonged fasting reduces IGF-1/PKA to promote hematopoietic-stem-cell-based regeneration and reverse immunosuppression. *Cell Stem Cell.* 2014; 14(6):810-823. https://www.ncbi.nlm.nih.gov/pubmed/24905167
This study in mice was performed to determine the effectiveness of fasting to counter the immunosuppression caused by chemotherapy. The article concluded that "our results indicate that cycles of an extreme dietary intervention represent a powerful means to modulate key regulators of cellular protection and tissue regeneration, but also provide a potential therapy to reverse or alleviate the immunosuppression or immunosenescence caused by chemotherapy treatment and aging."
This journal also published an editorial "Saying no to drugs: fasting protects hematopoietic stem cells from chemotherapy and aging" that comments on this study and research, and can be found here: https://www.ncbi.nlm.nih.gov/pmc/articles/PMC4278638/

Lee C, Raffaghello L, Brandhorst S, et al. Fasting cycles retard growth of tumors and sensitize a range of cancer cell types to chemotherapy. *Science Translational Medicine.* 2012; 124(4): 124ra27. https://stm.sciencemag.org/content/4/124/124ra27.short
A mouse study showing that cycles of fasting helped delay the progression of several tumor types, and that the combination of fasting and chemotherapy drugs was much more effective than either alone, and delayed the progression in a variety of tumors, including breast cancer and glioma (a type of brain cancer). This study is significant study because it raises the possibility that fasting could have the potential to help make traditional cancer therapies more effective, although there need to be studies done in human patients, not just mice.

National Institutes of Health: National Cancer Institute. Cancer Causes and Prevention – Cancer and Obesity.
https://www.cancer.gov/about-cancer/causes-prevention/risk/obesity/obesity-fact-sheet
This informational web site contains information and statistics about obesity and discusses the links between cancer and obesity. Specifically, the web site notes that there is consistent evidence that higher amounts of body fat are associated with increased risks of a number of cancers, including endometrial, esophageal, gastric cardia, liver, kidney, multiple myeloma, meningioma, pancreatic, colorectal, breast, gallbladder, thyroid, and ovarian.

Ohkuma, T, Peters, SAE, Woodward, M. Sex differences in the association between diabetes and cancer: a systematic review and meta-analysis of 121 cohorts including 20 million individuals and one million events. *Diabetologia.* 2018; 61:2140-2154.
https://doi.org/10.1007/s00125-018-4664-5
This phenomenal systematic review concluded that "diabetes is a risk factor for all-site cancer for both men and women, but the excess risk of cancer associated with diabetes is slightly greater for women than for men." Of note, they concluded that the evidence showed that diabetes conferred a significantly greater excess risk in women for oral, stomach, and kidney cancer.

Poff A, Koutnik AP, Egan KM, et al. Targeting the Warburg effect for cancer treatment: Ketogenic diets for management of glioma. Semin Cancer Biol. 2019; 56:135-148
https://www.sciencedirect.com/science/article/pii/S1044579X17301244
From the abstract: "This review will primarily focus on interventions to induce ketosis to target the glycolytic phenotype of many cancers, with specific application to secondary chemoprevention of low grade glioma – to halt the progression of lower grade tumors to more aggressive subtypes, as evidenced by reduction in validated intermediate endpoints of disease progression including clinical symptoms." This review of existing studies discusses the promise and potential of ketogenic therapies to slow and regress tumor development in glioma models by "targeting multiple signaling pathways that result in modulation of apoptosis, proliferation, inflammation, and related pathologies, relevant to progression in early stage disease to advanced cancers." They also note that research suggests that ketones do more than the originally described mechanism of reducing availability of glucose, and extends to working through multiple pathways of reducing inflammation, alterations in oxidative stress, enhancing anti-tumor immunity, altering gene expression, and sensitizing tumors to adjuvant therapies (thereby making traditional therapies more effective). But the authors conclude that due to a lack of definitive clinical data, more studies are

urgently needed to assess the potential of such non-toxic, cost-effective adjuvant ketogenic interventions in randomized controlled trials.

SECTION VIII

INFLAMMATION

Visser M, Bouter LM, McQuillan GM, et al. Elevated C-reactive protein levels in overweight and obese adults. *JAMA.* 1999; 282(22):2131-2135.
https://www.ncbi.nlm.nih.gov/pubmed/10591334
This paper studied 16,616 patients (a large study) and describes how fat tissue expresses and releases pro-inflammatory cytokine IL-6, which induces low-grade systemic inflammation in people with excess body fat. Inflammation was noted by elevated levels of C-reactive protein.

Goldberg EL, Dixit VD. Drivers of age-related inflammation and strategies for healthspan extension. *Immunol Rev.* 2015; 265(1):63-74.
https://www.ncbi.nlm.nih.gov/pmc/articles/PMC4400872/
This study discusses age related inflammation, and specifically how the NLRP3 inflammasome impacts aging in several organs in the body. It also notes that reduction of NLRP3 mediated inflammation prevents age-related insulin resistance, bone loss, cognitive decline, and frailty. It notes that therapies that reduce NLRP3 inflammation hold promise for reducing age-related diseases and may enhance lifespan.

Youm YH, Nguyen KY, Grant RW, et al. The ketone metabolite β-hydroxybutyrate blocks NLRP3 inflammasome-mediated inflammatory disease. *Nature Med.* 2015;21(3):263-9.
https://www.nature.com/articles/nm.3804
An excellent study published in *Nature Medicine*, one of the most prestigious medical scientific journals. A press release from Yale noted that "the researchers described how beta-hydroxybutyrate (BHB) directly inhibits NLRP3, which is part of a complex set of proteins called the inflammasome. The inflammasome drives the inflammatory response in several disorders including autoimmune diseases, type 2 diabetes, Alzheimer's disease, atherosclerosis, and auto-inflammatory disorders. These findings are important because endogenous metabolites like BHB that block the NLRP3 inflammasome could be relevant against many inflammatory diseases...."
The press release can be read in full here:
https://news.yale.edu/2015/02/16/anti-inflammatory-mechanism-dieting-and-fasting-revealed

Lamkanfi M, Dixit VM. *Inflammasomes and their roles in health and disease.* *Annu Rev Cell Dev Biol.* 2012; 28:137–161.
https://www.ncbi.nlm.nih.gov/pubmed/22974247
An excellent review that discusses inflammasomes, different inflammasome types, and their role in the inflammatory activity in autoinflammatory, autoimmune, and infectious diseases.

Sullivan PG, Rippy NA, Dorenbos K, et al. The Ketogenic diet increases mitochondrial uncoupling protein levels and activity. *Ann Neurology.* 2004;55(4):576-80.
https://www.ncbi.nlm.nih.gov/pubmed/15048898
This study showed that the ketogenic diet reduced reactive oxygen species (ROS) production, thereby exerting neuroprotective effects by diminishing ROS production through the process of enhanced activation of mitochondrial uncoupling protein by fatty acids.

Kim DY, Hao J, Liu R, et al. Inflammation-mediated memory dysfunction and effects of a ketogenic diet in a murine model of multiple sclerosis. *PLoS ONE.* 2012; 7(5):e35476.
https://www.ncbi.nlm.nih.gov/pubmed/22567104
This study investigated the effects of memory impairment and central nervous system inflammation and showed that mice fed the ketogenic diet improved their spatial memory and learning. It also showed inflammatory cytokines and production of reactive oxygen species (ROS) were suppressed by the ketogenic diet.

Sanada F, Taniyama Y, Muratsu J, et al. Source of chronic inflammation in aging. *Front Cardiovasc Med.* 2018; 5:12.
https://www.ncbi.nlm.nih.gov/pmc/articles/PMC5850851/
This article looks at the chronic pro-inflammatory status which is a pervasive feature of aging, called "inflammaging," and how chronic inflammation in aging is linked to a broad range of age-related diseases such as diabetes, atherosclerosis, and cancer. They discuss the factors and cellular pathways that lead to it: cell senescence (programmed cell death), cell debris, gut dysbiosis (dysfunction of the healthy gut bacteria/biome), immunosenescence, and pro-coagulation factor. In addition, they note the research showing that things like unbalanced diet and low level of sex hormones can contribute to aging. In addition, so can the accumulation of fat, as the accumulation of macrophages in visceral fat appears to be a major source of low-grade, persistent inflammation and insulin resistance in obese individuals. DNA damage caused by chronic low-level inflammation also contributes to aging.

Xia S, Zhang X, Zheng S, et al. An update on Inflamm-aging: mechanisms, prevention, and treatment. *J Immunol Res.* 2016; 8426874.
https://doi.org/10.1155/2016/8426874
https://www.ncbi.nlm.nih.gov/pmc/articles/PMC4963991/
This article notes that inflamm-aging is intensively associated with many age-related diseases such as Alzheimer's, atherosclerosis, type 2 diabetes, heart disease, Parkinson's disease, osteoporosis, macular degeneration, ALS, and cancer. The five states of inflamm-aging are low-grade, controlled,

asymptomatic, chronic, and systemic inflammation. Oxidative stress also plays a significant role and contributes not only to inflammation, but suppression of the immune system, and the combination of immunosenescence and inflamm-aging (immuno-inflamm-aging) plays a major role in the aging process.

Gkogkolou P, Bohm M. Advanced glycation end products: key players in skin aging? *Dermatoendocrinol.* 2012; 4(3):259-270.
https://www.ncbi.nlm.nih.gov/pmc/articles/PMC3583887/
Advanced glycation end products (AGEs) are non-enzymatic modifications of proteins or fats after exposure to sugars. Development of AGEs after food-browning and food processes was described in the 1960s and has been an extensive area of research in aging and diabetes. AGEs have been shown to accumulate in aged skin. Smoking also accelerates the formation of AGEs. Fried foods contain significantly higher amounts of AGEs than boiled or steamed foods. Dietary AGEs directly correlate to serum levels of AGEs and inflammatory markers in human subjects and are reactive molecules that are involved with inflammation, immune response, cell proliferation, gene expression and formation of reactive oxygen species (ROS). The authors discuss at length the impact of glycation in collagen, and its impact on skin aging. They also note that calorie restriction and various foods can improve or reduce AGE levels. Of importance to note is that levels of skin collagen glycation positively correlate with high blood glucose levels in diabetes.

Shen Y, Kapfhamer D, Minella M, et al. Bioenergetic state regulates innate inflammatory responses through the transcriptional co-repressor CtBP. *Nature Communications.* 2017; 8:624.
https://www.nature.com/articles/s41467-017-00707-0
This study looked at how changes in cellular glucose metabolism can influence cellular inflammatory responses, and describes how a ketogenic diet suppresses inflammation in brain cells in models of noninfectious states such as stroke and head trauma or traumatic brain injury.
An article describing it in less scientific terms can be found in the link below, noting that "the results may be applicable for other conditions besides brain-related inflammation. In patients with diabetes, excess glucose is linked to inflammation that can lead to heart disease."
https://www.ajpb.com/news/ketogenic-diet-suppresses-brain-inflammation

Fantuzzi G. Adiponectin and inflammation: consensus and controversy. *J Allergy Clin Immunol.* 2008; 121(2):326-30.
https://www.ncbi.nlm.nih.gov/pubmed/18061654
The protein adiponectin has been shown in multiple studies to demonstrate anti-inflammatory effects. This article discusses how adiponectin decreases with increasing visceral obesity, perpetuating low-level chronic inflammation in obese subjects, which increases insulin resistance and risk of

cardiovascular disease. Thus, low levels of adiponectin promote inflammation, creating a self-sustaining inflammatory loop.
However, in other non-obesity related diseases such as lupus, IBD, rheumatoid arthritis, type 1 diabetes, and cystic fibrosis, adiponectin levels are often elevated and have a pro-inflammatory effect. Thus, adiponectin is regulated in the opposite way and may exert the opposite effects in classic vs obesity-associated inflammatory conditions.

Yates T, Khunti K, Wilmot EG, et al. Self-reported sitting time and markers of inflammation, insulin resistance, and adiposity. *Am J Prev Med*. 2012; 42(1):1-7.
https://www.ajpmonline.org/article/S0749-3797(11)00731-8/abstract
An excellent article showing that time spent sitting correlated with increased biomarkers linked to chronic, low-grade inflammation and poor metabolic health, more so in women. This is significant because it supports the argument that sitting is damaging to metabolic health and contributes to inflammation – so get up frequently and move!

Dunstan DW, Salmon J, Healy GN, et al. Association of television viewing with fasting and 2-h postchallenge plasma glucose levels in adults without diagnosed diabetes. *Diabetes Care*. 2007; 30:516-22.
https://www.ncbi.nlm.nih.gov/pubmed/17327314
Similar to the previous article, this study tracked non-diabetic people watching TV (sitting, or engaging in sedentary time) and tested their fasting glucose and post-challenge glucose levels and insulin levels. These tests, when positive, are correlated with a higher risk of diabetes and cardiovascular disease. Not surprisingly, the sedentary TV watching time correlated positively with the higher glucose levels – and like the previously mentioned reference, it was notably more prominent in women. Again, this is significant because it reinforces the need to get people moving and active, rather than sitting around doing sedentary things like watching TV and sitting in front of a computer.

SECTION VIII

LUNG DISEASES AND COPD

Authors' Note: Chronic obstructive lung disease (COPD) is currently the 3rd leading killer globally, and is expected to continue to rise. It is a chronic disease with no cure, and progresses over time. It is characterized by airflow limitation, emphysema, and chronic infections like bronchitis and pneumonia. Interestingly, there is a lot of emerging research on how low-carb, high-fat and keto dieting can impact lung function and infection control and impact the airway epithelium and airway surface liquid.

Cornell K, Alam M, Lyden E, et al. Saturated fat intake is associated with lung function in individuals with airflow obstruction: results from NHANES 2007-2012. *Nutrients.* 2019; 11(2):317.
https://www.ncbi.nlm.nih.gov/pmc/articles/PMC6413158/
These researchers used data from the National Health and Nutrition Examination Surveys (NHANES) to look at the relationship between saturated fat intake and lung function, and found improvement in lung function is associated with increased saturated fat intake in individuals with COPD. This is significant because it has long been known that in hospitalized COPD patients, giving them a high fat diet improves gas exchange in the lung, and this study looked at the diet in patients in the general population and also found that it improved lung function.

Alessandro R, Gerardo B, Alessandra L, et al. Effects of twenty days of the ketogenic diet on metabolic and respiratory parameters in healthy subjects. *Lung.* 2015; 193:939-945.
https://link.springer.com/article/10.1007/s00408-015-9806-7
This study on 32 healthy subjects showed that following a ketogenic diet for only 20 days resulted in reduction in body mass, and the ketogenic diet group also showed significant reductions in carbon dioxide output and PETCO2 (end-tidal CO2) which may be beneficial for patients with respiratory insufficiency or respiratory failure.

Global Initiative for Chronic Obstructive Lung Disease (GOLD) 2019. Pocket guide to COPD diagnosis, management, and prevention. A guide for healthcare professionals. 2019 Edition.
https://goldcopd.org/wp-content/uploads/2018/11/GOLD-2019-POCKET-GUIDE-FINAL_WMS.pdf
A definitive set of guidelines for treating COPD. What's notable is there is pretty much ZERO guidance on nutrition, which is, sadly, something we see commonly in medical guidelines. This guideline focuses almost exclusively on diagnosis and pharmaceutical interventions with very little space devoted to non-pharmaceutical management.

Cui W, Zhang Z, Zhang P, et al. Nrf2 attenuates inflammatory response in COPD/emphysema: crosstalk with Wnt3a/B-catenin and AMPK pathways. *J Cell Mol Med.* 2018; 22(7):3514-3525.
https://www.ncbi.nlm.nih.gov/pmc/articles/PMC6010849/
This study looked at models of COPD, a chronic lung disease characterized by airflow limitations and abnormal inflammatory response. The authors showed that activation of the Nrf2 pathway mediated the protective effects lung inflammatory response during the development of COPD/emphysema.

Milder JB, Liang LP, Patel M. Acute oxidative stress and systemic Nrf2 activation by the ketogenic diet. *Neurobiol Dis.* 2010; 40(1):238-244.
https://www.ncbi.nlm.nih.gov/pubmed/20594978
This study showed that the ketogenic diet activates the Nrf2 pathway, which led to cellular adaptation, induction of protective proteins and helped reduce and eliminate oxidative stress.

Rahman I. Inflammation and the regulation of glutathione level in lung epithelial cells. *Antioxid Redox Signal.* 1999; 1(4):425-447.
https://www.ncbi.nlm.nih.gov/pubmed/11233143
Chronic inflammation is a hallmark of many inflammatory lung diseases. And reactive oxygen species are major causes of cell damage. Glutathione is a protective anti-oxidant in the lungs and plays a key role in regulating oxidant induced lung epithelial cell function. The authors of this paper stress the potential role for glutathione to alleviate lung oxidant stress, inflammation, and injury.
This study is important because it relates to the next study below.

Jarrett SG, Milder JB, Liang LP, Patel M. The ketogenic diet increases mitochondrial glutathione levels. *J Neurochem.* 2008; 106(3):1044-51
https://www.ncbi.nlm.nih.gov/pubmed/18466343/
This study showed that "the ketogenic diet up-regulates glutathione biosynthesis, enhances mitochondrial antioxidant status, and protects mtDNA from oxidant-induced damage."
So, the previous study above this one showed how glutathione helps protect the lungs and alleviates inflammation and lung injury, and this study shows that the ketogenic diet upregulated glutathione synthesis.

Baker EH, Baines DL. Airway glucose homeostasis: A new target in the prevention and treatment of pulmonary infection. *Chest.* 2018; 153(2):507-514.
https://www.ncbi.nlm.nih.gov/pubmed/28610911
This study discussed the role of glucose concentration in airway surface liquid in the airways. Elevated airway surface liquid glucose levels allow proliferation of certain types of bacterial infections in the lung, whereas

lower levels appear to limit bacterial growth, and so this study suggests that lower glucose levels may be a target to help prevent and fight lung infections, especially in inflammatory diseases such as COPD. It also reinforces the need to manage blood glucose levels, especially in diseases like diabetes, which seem to make people more prone to lung infections.

Thaker SK, Ch'ng J, Christofk HR. Viral hijacking of cellular metabolism. *BMC Biology.* 2019; 17:59.
https://bmcbiol.biomedcentral.com/articles/10.1186/s12915-019-0678-9
This study looks at how viruses use cellular metabolism to proliferate, and like cancer, many types of viruses are characterized by large upregulation of glycolysis. This implies that low-carb and ketogenic diets may support anti-viral immune responses.

MULTIPLE SCLEROSIS

Choi IY, Piccio L, Childress P, et al. A diet mimicking fasting promotes regeneration and reduces autoimmunity and multiple sclerosis symptoms. *Cell Rep. 2016*; 15(10):2136-2146.
https://www.ncbi.nlm.nih.gov/pubmed/27239035
This study tested periodic 3-day cycles of a fasting mimicking diet (FMD). Highlights of the study were that FMD reduced pro-inflammatory cytokines and increased corticosterone levels, FMD suppressed autoimmunity be inducing lymphocyte apoptosis, FMD promoted regeneration of oligodendrocyte in multiple MS models, and that FMD (or a ketogenic diet) is a safe, feasible, and potentially effective treatment for MS patients.

Storoni M, Plant GT. The therapeutic potential of the ketogenic diet in treating progressive multiple sclerosis. *Mult Scler Int.* 2015; 2015:68128.
https://www.ncbi.nlm.nih.gov/pmc/articles/PMC4709725/
This study challenged the notion that MS is purely an inflammatory disease, and focused on the significant neurodegenerative component responsible for the progression of MS. Most MS cases are relapsing and remitting (called RRMS), meaning they recur but typically resolve with conservative management; whereas in 15% of cases, the disease presents with a gradual and progressive loss of neurologic function that does not recover (called PPMS). The authors describe various components of MS that are neurodegenerative in nature, including mitochondrial dysfunction, and how the ketogenic diet can help counter those issues.
The authors conclude that the ketogenic diet has the potential to treat the degenerative component of progressive MS on the basis of the fact that progressive MS is a neurodegenerative disease; mitochondrial dysfunction resulting in reduced ATP production that is a hallmark of the disease; and the ketogenic diet increases ATP production, promotes mitochondrial biogenesis, and bypasses the mitochondrial dysfunction (*ie,* ketones are more easily utilized for energy).

SECTION VIII

DERMATOLOGY

Fomin DA, McDaniel B, Crane J. The promising potential role of ketones in inflammatory dermatologic disease: a new frontier in treatment research. *J Dermatol Treatment.* 2017; 28(6):484-487.
https://www.tandfonline.com/doi/abs/10.1080/09546634.2016.1276259
This study looked at the literature for known causes of inflammation in dermatologic diseases and correlated that with suggested mechanisms of anti-inflammatory activity of ketones and a ketogenic state in the human body. They found that "ketones modulate the NLRP3 inflammasome, augment anti-oxidation against reactive oxygen species through various direct and indirect means, and my influence mTOR activity, which are all involved in inflammatory dermatologic diseases"...."This evidence shows that ketones and the ketogenic diet may have a promising role in the dermatologist's disease treatment repertoire."

POLYCYSTIC OVARY SYNDROME (PCOS)

Mavropoulos JC, Yancy WS, Hepburn J, Westman E. The effects of a low-carbohydrate, ketogenic diet on the polycystic ovary syndrome: a pilot study. *Nutr Metab.* 2005; 2:35.
https://www.ncbi.nlm.nih.gov/pmc/articles/PMC1334192/
Polycystic ovary syndrome (PCOS) is an endocrine disorder affecting women of reproductive age and is associated with obesity, hyperinsulinemia, insulin resistance, and hormone imbalances. This study investigated patients for 6 months using a low carb keto diet in overweight and obese women with PCOS. Not surprisingly (to us!) there was significant improvement in weight, percentage of free testosterone, LH/FSH ratio, and fasting insulin. In addition, there were decreases noted in insulin, glucose, and A1c although the researchers did not consider them statistically significant. Two women became pregnant during the study despite previous infertility problems.

Goss AM, Chandler-Laney PC, Ovalle F, et al. Effects of a eucalorid reduced-carbohydrate diet on body composition and fat distribution in women with PCOS. *Metabolism.* 2014; 63(10):1257-1264.
https://www.sciencedirect.com/science/article/pii/S0026049514002108
In women with PCOS, eating a low-carb diet was shown not only to cause fat loss, but to preferentially lose fat from areas that were metabolically harmful, such as subcutaneous belly fat, intra-abdominal visceral fat, and thigh fat. It also showed that eating a high-carb diet promoted fat gain and less lean muscle.

Sorensen LB, Soe M, Halker KH, et al. Effects of increased dietary protein-to-carbohydrate ratios in women with polycystic ovary syndrome. *Am J Clin Nutrition.* 2012; 95(1):39-48
https://academic.oup.com/ajcn/article/95/1/39/4576669?ncid=txtlnkusaolp00000618
This study showed that replacing carbs with protein (low-carb, high protein) improved weight loss, and also improved glucose metabolism that was unrelated to the weight loss. Again, carbs seem to exacerbate PCOS.

Mavropoulos JC, Yancy WS, Hepburn J, Westman EC. The effects of a low-carbohydrate, ketogenic diet on the polycystic ovary syndrome: A pilot study. *Nutr Metab.* 2005; 2:35
https://www.ncbi.nlm.nih.gov/pubmed/16359551
Polycystic ovary syndrome is the most common endocrine disorder affecting women of reproductive age and is associated with obesity, hyperinsulinemia, and insulin resistance. So the researchers put women on a low-carb ketogenic diet for 6 months. Results showed that the low-carb ketogenic diet

led to significant improvement in weight, free testosterone, LH/FSH ratio, and fasting insulin levels. Keto for the win!

Tata B, El Houda Mimouni N, Barbotin A-L, et al. Elevated prenatal anti-Mullerian hormone reprograms the fetus and induces polycystic ovary syndrome in adulthood. *Nature Medicine.* 2018; 24:834-846. https://www.nature.com/articles/s41591-018-0035-5
Women with PCOS often have difficulty conceiving. However, it's also important to note that one of the hallmarks of PCOS is hormone imbalance. In PCOS, there is often a surplus of Anti-Mullerian hormone, and this study looked at how excess AMH during pregnancy may cause over-masculinization in a mouse fetus and lead to adult PCOS. This supports the hypothesis that PCOS can be passed down, although it was a mouse study, not a human study.

MIGRAINES

Di Lorenzo C, Coppola G, Sirianni G, et al. Migraine improvement during short lasting ketogenesis: a proof-of-concept study. *Eur J Neurol.* 2015; 22(1):170-177.
https://www.ncbi.nlm.nih.gov/pubmed/25156013
This study looked at women with migraines and either put them on a 1-month keto diet followed by 5 months of a standard diet, or a 6-month standard diet. The group on the keto diet showed significant reductions in attack frequency, number of days with headaches, and migraine medicine intake. Once they went off the keto diet, the frequency began to increase, but still remained less than baseline up to month 6. They concluded that the ketogenic diet helped migraines because of its ability to enhance mitochondrial energy metabolism in the brain, and counteract neural inflammation.

Zaeem Z, Zhou L, Dilli E. Headaches: a review of the role of dietary factors Curr Neurol Neurosci Rep. 2016; 16(5):101.
https://www.ncbi.nlm.nih.gov/pubmed/27714637
This review discussed dietary triggers most commonly reported by patients with a variety of headaches, particularly those with migraines. The authors noted that some foods trigger headache within an hour while others develop within 12 hours after ingestion. Alcohol (especially red wine and beer), chocolate, caffeine, dairy products such as aged cheese, food preservatives with nitrates and nitrites, monosodium glutamate (MSG), and artificial sweeteners such as aspartame have all been studied as migraine triggers in the past. This review focused the evidence linking these compounds to headache and examined the prevalence of these triggers from prior population-based studies. Recent literature surrounding headache related to fasting and weight loss as well as elimination diets based on serum food antibody testing were also summarized to help physicians recommend low-risk, non-pharmacological adjunctive therapies for patients with debilitating headaches.

Barbanti P, Fofi L, Aurilia C, et al. Ketogenic diet in migraine: rationale, findings and perspectives, Neurol Sci. 2017; 38(5)(Suppl 1):111-115.
https://www.ncbi.nlm.nih.gov/pubmed/28527061
This review of the literature discussed how clinical data on 150 patients suggest that the ketogenic diet provides rapid onset effective prophylaxis for episodic and chronic migraines. The authors conclude that keto would contribute to the body's ability to restore brain excitability and metabolism, and to counteract neuro-inflammation in migraines.

SECTION VIII

Nakanishi Y, Tsuneyama K, Fujimoto M, et al. Monosodium glutamate (MSG): A villain and promoter of liver inflammation and dysplasia. *J Autoimmun.* 2008; 30(1-2):42-50.
https://www.ncbi.nlm.nih.gov/pubmed/18178378
This study highlighted the potential health effects of MSG, showing that it is associated with development of chronic inflammation, obesity, type 2 diabetes, and nonalcoholic steatohepatitis (NASH), which has been increasing in incidence in the westernized world. The authors called for the safety profile of MSG to be re-examined and potentially withdrawn from the food chain.

Di Lorenzo C, Coppola G, Sirianni G, Pierelli F. Short term improvement of migraine headaches during ketogenic diet: a prospective observational study in a dietician clinical setting. *J Headache Pain.* 2013; 14(suppl 1):P219.
https://www.ncbi.nlm.nih.gov/pmc/articles/PMC3620251/
Preliminary report of a previously cited article. Authors put migraine suffers on a ketogenic diet and saw headache frequency and migraine medication use drop significantly. Their findings support the role of the ketogenic diet in migraine treatment.

EXERCISE AND ATHLETIC PERFORMANCE

Volek JS, Freidenreich DJ, Saenz C, et al. Metabolic characteristics of keto-adapted ultra-endurance runners. *Metabolism.* 2016; 65(3):100-110
https://www.sciencedirect.com/science/article/pii/S0026049515003340
This study compared highly trained ultra-endurance athletes who ate a high-carb diet vs a low carb ketogenic diet. The keto-adapted athletes saw very high rates of fat oxidation, whereas muscle glycogen utilization and repletion patterns during and after a 3-hour run were similar – meaning fat was readily used for energy. This is significant because fat provides more energy per gram than glucose.

Zajac A, Poprzecki S, Maszczyk A, et al. The effects of a ketogenic diet on exercise metabolism and physical performance in off-road cyclists. *Nutrients.* 2014; 6(7):2493-2508.
https://www.ncbi.nlm.nih.gov/pmc/articles/PMC4113752/
This small study in 8 off-road cyclists showed that following a ketogenic diet improved body mass and body composition, lipid and lipoprotein profiles, and significant increase in maximal oxygen uptake (VO2max) and oxygen uptake at lactate threshold (VO2LT). The authors attribute this most likely to increased energy yield from fat oxidation. It was also notable that the respiratory exchange ratio improved, something that other studies have shown. Creatine kinase and lactate dehydrogenase were also lower during some portions of the study in the keto group. In addition, heart rate and oxygen uptake were higher at rest and during the earlier stages of exercise with the ketogenic diet vs a mixed diet, but were lower during the last state at maximal intensity, showing that for serious endurance athletes, even if fat adapted, they may need additional fuel from carbohydrates in order to maintain maximal intensity in late stages of activity.

Brinkworth GD, Noakes M, Clifton PM, Buckley JD. Effects of a low carbohydrate weight loss diet on exercise capacity and tolerance in obese subjects. *Obesity.* 2009; 17(10):1916-23.
https://www.ncbi.nlm.nih.gov/pubmed/19373224
Full text: https://onlinelibrary.wiley.com/doi/full/10.1038/oby.2009.134
This study on obese individuals put them on either a low carb or high carb diet, and tested a number of parameters. Not surprisingly, the group on the low-carb diet lost significantly more weight than the group on the high-carb diet. In the end, there were no significant differences between the groups on exercise capacity and other measures such as grip strength. However, it's hard to say the study proves one way or another whether a low carb diet would impact athletic performance because the study was done in obese individuals, not conditioned athletes.

SECTION VIII

Phinney SD, Horton ES, Sims EA, et al. Capacity for moderate exercise in obese subjects after adaptation to a hypocaloric, ketogenic diet. *J Clin Invest.* 1980; 66(5):1152-1161.
https://www.ncbi.nlm.nih.gov/pubmed/7000826
This early seminal study by Phinney and colleagues looked at the capacity for moderate endurance exercise and change in metabolic fuel usage during the adaptation to a ketogenic diet. It showed that prolonged ketosis results in fat-adaption (keto-adaption), which results in fat being used as fuel.
A very key piece of early science supporting keto as a way to change your body's fuel source from carbs to fat and ketones!

Cox PJ, Kirk T, Ashmore T, et al. Nutritional ketosis alters fuel preference and thereby exercise endurance in athletes. *Cell Metab.* 2016; 24(2):256-268.
https://www.ncbi.nlm.nih.gov/pubmed/27475046
This study was performed on athletes using a ketone ester drink supplement to achieve nutritional ketosis. The article discusses how 5 separate studies of 39 high-performance athletes showed how this state of ketosis improves physical endurance. Ketosis decreased muscle glycolysis and blood lactate concentrations, as well as intramuscular triacylglycerol oxidation during exercise, even then glycogen was present and carbohydrates were consumed. The findings showed that the body will preferentially use ketones even when other fuel sources are present in the body, and that the use of ketones enhances endurance and performance times.
Full text of the article available here: https://www.sciencedirect.com/science/article/pii/S1550413116303552

Urbain P, Strom L, Morawski L, et al. Impact of a 6-week non-energy-restricted ketogenic diet on physical fitness, body composition, and biochemical parameters in healthy adults. *Nutr Metab.* 2017; 14:17.
https://www.ncbi.nlm.nih.gov/pmc/articles/PMC5319032/
This study of 42 people put them on a 6-week ketogenic diet and measured multiple physical performance parameters. Overall, there was a slight decrease in exercise endurance performance but there were also positive changes in body composition and handgrip strength. Some of the results were inconsistent and conflicted with the results of other previously published studies. The study did call for study of a longer ketogenic diet regimen than only 6 weeks.

Volek JS, Noakes T, Phinney SD. Rethinking fat as a fuel for endurance exercise. *Eur J Sports Science.* 2015; 15(1):13-20.
https://www.tandfonline.com/doi/abs/10.1080/17461391.2014.959564
This article by three of the fathers of low-carb nutrition, ketones and athletic performance highlights how fat-adaptation through ketogenic nutrition could extend human physical and mental performance beyond current expectation. They propose that the fueling shift from glucose and glycogen to fatty acids and ketones as primary fuels could be of benefit for athletes.

Harvey KL, Holcomb LE, Kolwicz Jr., SC. Ketogenic diets and exercise performance. *Nutrients.* 2019; 11(10):2296. https://www.ncbi.nlm.nih.gov/pmc/articles/PMC6835497/
This article provides a nice review of the literature, and highlights some of the controversial and sometimes conflicting results of studies on the keto diet and ketone supplementation on exercise performance, and they also tackle the topic of ketones as a therapy for heart dysfunction (odd that they tackled that in an article primarily about exercise performance). All in all, a great read, although in our opinion, they miss some obvious conclusions.
[Comment from Steve and Dr. Lori: Although some studies show that ketosis can help certain, but not all, aspects of exercise performance, and other studies do not, what is very obvious is that there are almost no long-term studies in the exercise performance area. Almost all the studies reviewed and cited in this review are looking at athletes on a ketogenic diet for 4 weeks, 1 month, or 6 weeks. In our opinion, this is hardly a long enough timeframe to allow full keto and fat adaptation and for a trained athlete to make adjustments to their training that would maximize a new way of eating and fueling one's body. The other thing that's obvious is that in high-intensity situations, there is a need for glucose or glycogen and that for many athletes, a dual fuel nutrition plan (combined with ketone supplementation), especially during competitive events, may be necessary (we want to see THAT studied!).]

KETONE SUPPLEMENTATION

Kovacs Z, D'Agostino DP, Diamond D, et al. Therapeutic potential of exogenous ketone supplement induced ketosis in the treatment of psychiatric disorders: review of current literature. *Front Psychiatry.* 2019; 10:363.
https://www.ncbi.nlm.nih.gov/pubmed/31178772
Emerging evidence from many studies suggests that exogenous ketone supplements generate rapid and sustained nutritional ketosis and metabolic changes that may evoke potential therapeutic effects in cases of central nervous system (CNS) disorders, including psychiatric diseases. This review looked at studies on depression, schizophrenia, anxiety, autism spectrum disorders, bipolar disorders, and ADHD.
Ketone supplementation elevates blood levels of the ketone bodies D-β-hydroxybutyrate (βHB, also commonly referred to as BHB), acetoacetate (AcAc), and acetone. The result of downstream cellular and molecular changes is a reduction in the pathophysiology associated with various psychiatric disorders. The authors conclude that supplement-induced nutritional ketosis leads to metabolic changes and improvements, for example, in mitochondrial function and inflammatory processes, and suggest that development of specific adjunctive ketogenic protocols for psychiatric diseases should be actively pursued.

Taylor MK, Swerdlow RH, Sullivan DK. Dietary neuroketotherapeutics for Alzheimer's disease: an evidence update and the potential role for diet quality. *Nutrients.* 2019; 11(8):E1910.
https://www.ncbi.nlm.nih.gov/pubmed/31443216
Free full text: https://www.mdpi.com/2072-6643/11/8/1910/htm
This review of the literature and evidence noted that a consistent hallmark of Alzheimer's disease is reduced brain glucose utilization, but evidence suggests that ketone metabolism remains unimpaired. Therefore, there is great interest in the potential value of ketone-inducing therapies for the treatment of Alzheimer's. This review looks at the ketogenic diet, fasting, exogenous ketone supplementation, and MCT supplementation. Although it cites numerous studies showing promise, it calls for more trials to secure an evidence base that is strong enough to make sound recommendations.

Fortier M, Castellano CA, Croteau E, et al. A ketogenic drink improves brain energy and some measures of cognition in mild cognitive impairment. *Alzheimers Dement* 2019; 15(5):625-634.
https://www.ncbi.nlm.nih.gov/pubmed/31027873
This blinded, randomized, placebo-controlled study looked at 52 subjects who were given a ketone drink or a placebo drink (no ketones) and tested cognitive performance at baseline vs 6 months later. Results showed that brain ketone metabolism increased by 230% in the group receiving the

ketone drink. Measures of episodic memory, language, executive function, and processing speed improved in the ketone drink group vs baseline. This is significant because it showed that keeping ketones elevated into a therapeutic range helped brain function, even in people with cognitive impairment.

Csilla A, Kovacs Z, Juhasz G, et al. Exogenous ketone supplements reduce anxiety-related behavior in Sprague-Dawley and Wistar Albino Glaxo/ Rijswijk Rats. *Front Mol Neurosci.* 2016; 9:137.
https://www.ncbi.nlm.nih.gov/pmc/articles/PMC5138218/
This study by top ketone researcher Dominic D'Agostino and colleagues was initiated because of the proven effectiveness of nutritional ketosis for seizure disorders and neurologic disorders. They sought to determine the effects of exogenous ketone supplementation on anxiety-related behavior in rats. They tested both ketone esters and racemic ketone salts containing the ketone metabolite beta-hydroxybutyrate (BHB). The study showed that exogenous ketone supplementation elevated BHB levels in both animal models and also decreased anxiety-related behaviors, concluding that ketone supplementation may provide a promising anti-anxiety therapy by inducing ketosis.

Kesl SL, Poff AM, Ward NP, et al. Effects of exogenous ketone supplementation on blood ketone, glucose, triglyceride, and lipoprotein levels in Sprague-Dawley rats. *Nutr Metab.* 2016; 13:9.
https://nutritionandmetabolism.biomedcentral.com/articles/10.1186/s12986-016-0069-y
In this study, the researchers measured the effects of 28 days of administered supplemental ketones in rats, and showed that the ketone administration elevated blood levels of the ketone metabolite beta-hydroxybutyrate (BHB) without any dietary restrictions, and reduced blood glucose levels. This is significant because it showed that even when eating carbohydrates, taking an exogenous ketone supplement put blood ketone levels in a therapeutic range. It also showed application for lowering blood glucose levels, which may prove to have potential benefits for diabetic patients.

Poff AM, Rho JM, D'Agostino DP. Ketone administration for seizure disorders: History and rationale for ketone esters and metabolic alternatives. *Front Neurosci.* 2019; 13:1041.
https://www.ncbi.nlm.nih.gov/pmc/articles/PMC6803688/
This article discusses the use of the ketogenic diet as a proven effective treatment for epilepsy and certain seizure disorders. However, adhering to a strict diet is not always easy and feasible and compliance with it is an issue. Therefore, they discuss the science behind the use of exogenous ketone supplementation to elevate blood levels of the ketone bodies beta-hydroxybutyrate and acetoacetate. They note that elevating these ketone bodies in the blood has been shown to have an anti-seizure effect in animal

models, and so they call for clinical trials in humans because this represents a clinically viable potential treatment of epilepsy and other seizure disorders.

Hashim SA, VanItallie TB. Ketone body therapy: from the ketogenic diet to the oral administration of ketone ester. *J Lipid Res.* 2014; 55(9):1818-1826. https://www.ncbi.nlm.nih.gov/pmc/articles/PMC4617348/
This is an excellent review of the literature that discusses ketones, ketosis, and the ketogenic diet, as well as exogenous ketone ester supplements. They also discuss the potential therapeutic uses of ketones including Alzheimer's disease, Parkinson's disease, and epilepsy. At the time of publication of this article in 2014, ketone supplements were barely available and quite new conceptually – and the authors note their therapeutic potential and actually call for clinical trials using FDA approved ketone esters.

LONGEVITY AND CALORIE RESTRICTION / FASTING

Veech RL, Bradshaw PC, Clarke K, et al. Ketone bodies mimic the life-extending properties of caloric restriction. *IUBMB Life.* 2017; 69(5):305-314. https://iubmb.onlinelibrary.wiley.com/doi/10.1002/iub.1627
The extension of lifespan by calorie restriction has been seen in a variety of species from yeast to worms to primates. In this critical review, the authors propose that life span extension produced by caloric restriction can be duplicated by the metabolic changes induced by ketosis. They note the mechanisms for this, which is tied to decreased signaling through the insulin/insulin-like growth factor receptor signaling pathway. They also note that an effective method for combating free radical damage occurs though the metabolism of ketone bodies. They also note that supplementing with ketones also decreases circulating glucose and insulin leading to that same decreased insulin signaling pathway. They noted especially that the addition of the ketone body beta-hydroxybutyrate extended the lifespan of *C. elegans* nematodes. This all culminates in the suggestion of new lines of research in humans around ketosis and ketones in aging and age-related disorders.

Moreno CL, Mobbs CV. Epigenetic mechanisms underlying lifespan and age-related effects of dietary restriction and the ketogenic diet. M*ol Cell Endocrinol.* 2017; 455:33-40.
https://www.sciencedirect.com/science/article/abs/pii/S0303720716304828
This article discusses aging as the central risk factor for major diseases such as cancer, neurodegeneration, and heart disease. It reviews the evidence that dietary restriction delays aging associated with epigenetics, and discusses how ketogenic diets may entail similar protective epigenetic mechanisms.

Choi Y, Lee C, Longo VD. Nutrition and fasting mimicking diets in the prevention and treatment of autoimmune diseases and immunosenescence. *Mol Cellular Endocrinol.* 2017; 455:4-12.
https://www.sciencedirect.com/science/article/abs/pii/S0303720717300552
This article reviews the literature behind dietary restriction and fasting and how they decrease immunosenescence (programmed cell death in the immune system), as well as how fasting mimicking diets promote anti-inflammatory effects and alleviate or reverse autoimmune disorders in mice and possibly humans.

Bruss MD, Khambatta CF, Ruby MA, et al. Calorie restriction increases fatty acid synthesis and whole body fat oxidation rates. *Am J Physiol Endocrinol Metab.* 2010; 298(1):E108-E116.
https://www.ncbi.nlm.nih.gov/pmc/articles/PMC4056782/

SECTION VIII

An interesting study in mice that looked at how when calories are restricted, the body cycles between synthesizing fatty acids (breaking them down into molecules used for essential substances in our cells, signaling, hormone production, and other functions) to oxidizing them (using them for energy). The calorie restricted mice oxidized 4 times as much fat per day as the mice who ate as much as they wanted, mostly from adipose tissue (body fat). So the takeaway is that calorie restriction (fasting) can really help move your body into a fat burning state, and this increased synthesis of fatty acids may play a key role in quelling oxidative damage and disease risk.

Speakman JR, Mitchell SE. Caloric restriction. *Mol Aspects Med.* 2011; 32(3):159-221.
https://www.ncbi.nlm.nih.gov/pubmed/21840335?dopt=Abstract
This review discusses research supporting the theories and behind calorie restriction as a way to extend lifespan, quality of life, and reduce development of diseases such as cancer, neurodegenerative disorders, autoimmune disease, cardiovascular disease, and type 2 diabetes. They also note the profound impact calorie restriction has on reducing blood glucose and insulin levels, and shifting the metabolism from burning carbs to burning fat for energy. They also note how calorie restriction reduces oxidative stress and enhances autophagy (cellular debris cleanup).

Roberts MN, Wallace MA, Tomilov AA, et al. A ketogenic diet extends longevity and healthspan in adult mice. *Cell Metab.* 2017; 26(3):539-546.e5.
https://www.ncbi.nlm.nih.gov/pmc/articles/PMC5609489/
Full text: https://www.cell.com/cell-metabolism/fulltext/S1550-4131(17)30490-4
In this study, mice were given either a ketogenic, a low-carb, or a standard control diet and allowed to live out their lifespan. The ketogenic diet group had significantly increased median lifespan compared to control group and decreased tumor incidence. In the older mice, only those consuming a ketogenic diet displayed preservation of physiologic function and memory.

Meidenbauer JJ, Ta N, Seyfried TN. Influence of a ketogenic diet, fish oil, and calorie restriction on plasma metabolites and lipids in C57BL/6J mice. *Nutr Metab.* 2014; 11:23.
https://www.ncbi.nlm.nih.gov/pmc/articles/PMC4047269/
A very interesting study that compared 3 different diets (ketogenic diet, standard diet, and standard diet + fish oil supplements) intended to drop body weight by 20% in mice. This study had some surprising results including showing the ketogenic diet group had higher glucose levels – this may have been because of a high level of gluconeogenesis. But the authors' conclusion was that the biomarkers of health could be improved when diets are consumed in restricted amounts. They also got some results that supported the idea that all calories are not equal.

FIBER

Wanders AJ, van den Borne JJ, de Graaf C, et al. Effects of dietary fibre on subjective appetite, energy intake, and body weight: a systematic review of randomized controlled trials. *Obes Rev.* 2011; 12(9):724-739.
https://www.ncbi.nlm.nih.gov/pubmed/21676152
This systematic review looked at randomized controlled trials on fiber, and their ability to reduce subjective appetite, energy intake and body weight. But different types of fiber may affect these outcomes differently. Their review sought to look at differences between fiber based on its viscosity, solubility, and fermentability. Their analysis did show differences based on the characteristics of the fiber. Fiber characterized as being more viscous (pectins, B-glucans, and guar gum) reduced appetite more than the less viscous fibers, and that also applied to acute energy intake. Effects on energy and body weight were actually fairly small.

Klosterbuer A, Sanders L, Potter S, et al. A blend of soluble fiber and resistant starch promotes feelings of fullness in humans. *FASEB J.* 2010; 24(suppl 1):220.4.
https://www.fasebj.org/doi/abs/10.1096/fasebj.24.1_supplement.220.4
This abstract was presented at the 2010 FASEB meeting and showed that soluble fiber caused greater feelings of fullness and reduced glucose and insulin AUC.

Krishnamurthy VM, Wei G, Baird BC, et al. High dietary fiber intake is associated with decreased inflammation and all-cause mortality in patients with chronic kidney disease. *Kidney Int.* 2012; 81(3):300-306.
https://www.ncbi.nlm.nih.gov/pubmed/22012132
This study reviewed data from the National Health and Nutrition Examination Survey III to determine whether fiber intake was associated with better health outcomes in kidney disease patients. Interestingly, high fiber was not associated with reduced mortality in patients without kidney disease, but was associated with lower mortality in those with kidney disease. It also showed an association with decreased inflammation.

Parnell JA, Reimer RA. Prebiotic fiber modulation of the gut microbiota improves risk factors for obesity and the metabolic syndrome. *Gut Microbes.* 2012; 3(1):29-34.
https://www.ncbi.nlm.nih.gov/pmc/articles/PMC3827018/
These researches studied the response to a prebiotic diet on the gut microbiota, body composition and obesity related risk factors in rats, since imbalance in gut microbes is present in a number of metabolic disorders. The prebiotic diet caused positive changes in the gut microbiota that correlated with the same balance seen in leaner phenotypes.

SECTION VIII

Yunsheng M, Griffith JA, Chasan-Taber L, et al. Association between dietary fiber and serum C-reactive protein. *Am J Clin Nutr.* 2006; 83(4):760-766. https://www.ncbi.nlm.nih.gov/pmc/articles/PMC1456807/
C-reactive protein is a marker of acute inflammation and has been identified as an independent predictor of future cardiovascular disease and diabetes. This study of 524 patients looked at the relationship between fiber intake and CRP levels, and the results suggest that dietary fiber may be protective against high CRP.

Lattimer JM, Haub MD. Effects of dietary fiber and its components on metabolic health. *Nutrients.* 2010; 2(12):1266-1289. https://www.ncbi.nlm.nih.gov/pmc/articles/PMC3257631/
This excellent review of the literature describes the definition and functions of fiber, and looks at the blend of bioactive compounds in fiber such as resistant starches, vitamins, minerals, phytochemicals, and antioxidants and how they correlate with different health parameters. Epidemiologic and clinical studies have demonstrated that dietary fiber consumption is inversely related to obesity, type 2 diabetes, cancer (especially colorectal, small intestine, oral, larynx, and breast), and cardiovascular disease. However, the studies on independent fractions such as arabinoxylan, inulin, pectin, bran, cellulose, beta-glucan and resistant starches have been inconsistent. The reviewers sought to review literature and evidence on these independent fractions, as well as discussing how fiber is fermented and produces short chain fatty acids, which are also linked to various health parameters. A great overall literature review and discussion of fiber and its components and their impact on health and disease.

AUTHOR PROFILES

Lori Shemek, PhD, CNC

Lori Shemek, PhD, CNC is a leading fat cell researcher, health expert, weight loss expert, keynote speaker, award-winning author and recognized authority on inflammation and its role in weight loss, preventing disease and optimizing health. Dr. Shemek is the bestselling author of three books: *'How To Fight FATflammation!' (HarperCollins), "Fire-Up Your Fat Burn!'* and *'The Beginner's Guide to Intermittent Fasting.*

Dr. Lori Shemek has been featured in or on CBS The Doctors TV, ABC TV show Good Morning Texas health expert, has been featured on CNN, Time, NPR and Fox News, The Ricki Lake Show, Oprah.com, Dr. Oz's Good Life Magazine, NBC Today, Health, Shape, Woman's Day, Prevention, Redbook, Ladies Home Journal, Men's Health, The Huffington Post, Closer Magazine, Yahoo.com, Fitness Magazine, EveryDay Health, Eat This, Not That!, Bustle, Consumer Health Digest and numerous others, including national syndicated radio such as Fox News Radio.

Dr. Shemek is known as "The Inflammation Terminator." She has made it her mission to educate the public on the toxic effects of certain foods and lifestyle choices and how they create inflammation in the body resulting in weight gain and poor health.

The Huffington Post has recognized Dr. Shemek twice as one of the *Top Health and Fitness Experts* alongside such names as Dr. Oz and David Zinczenko author of 'Eat This, Not That!' and the Huffington Post has also recognized her as one of the *Top Diet and Nutrition Experts.*

Dr. Shemek holds a Doctorate in Psychology; she is a Certified Nutritional Consultant and a Certified Life Coach.

Visit www.drlorishemek.com to find out more about her books, coaching services, recommended products, and availability as a speaker at your next event!

Follow on twitter @LoriShemek and Instagram @DrLoriShemek and facebook @DrLoriShemek

Listen to "This Podcast Burns Fat" https://thispodcastburnsfat.libsyn.com/

Steve Welch, CFNC

Steve Welch is known as a fitness, nutrition, fat loss, and ketogenic expert who digs into scientific medical research to learn and coach about cutting edge nutritional concepts, fitness and athletic performance techniques, and refutes myths and misinformation, as well as disproven dogma.

Steve is the former publisher of the world renowned medical journal *CHEST,* and held multiple key roles at the American College of Chest Physicians during his 25 year career with the medical education organization, which culminated with him serving as its Executive Vice President and CEO. He also served as the Executive Vice President of the CHEST Foundation, its philanthropic arm.

He enjoys educating people and has extensive experience as a speaker at global educational events in multiple topic areas. Contact him for availability as a speaker at your upcoming event.

Steve is a National Exercise and Sports Trainers Association (NESTA) certified Fitness Nutrition Coach, and has been using and experimenting with low-carb and ketogenic nutrition and ketone supplementation for the past 6 years. He worked in the 1980s as a fitness trainer and competed as an amateur bodybuilder. His background in training and diet as well as fat loss and muscle hypertrophy has provided him with the knowledge and skills to educate others on optimal nutrition and exercise strategies to achieve better health and quality of life.

He served as editor of the book *Get Fit, Lean and Keep Your Day Job: A Transformation Guide for Any Body* by JD Griffin.

A lifelong scuba diver since the age of 15, Steve relaxes by diving with large sharks. He also has an affinity for rescuing great Danes, especially deaf ones.

Visit my web site at www.ketosteve.net
Follow me on twitter @ketosteve

Made in the USA
Columbia, SC
30 December 2020